Take Two Chocolates
and Call Me
in the Morning

Take Two Chocolates

Chocolates

and Call Me in the Morning

12 Semi-Practical Solutions for the Really Busy Woman

Emily Watts

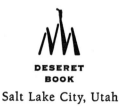

DESERET BOOK

Salt Lake City, Utah

Library of Congress Cataloging-in-Publication Data

Watts, Emily.
  Take two chocolates and call me in the morning / Emily Watts.
      p.   cm.
  ISBN 1-57008-903-5 (Paperback)
  1. Mothers—Life skills guides.   2. Wives—Life skills guides.   3. Stress management for women.   4. Women—Conduct of life.   5. Christian life—Mormon authors.   I. Title.
  HQ759.W356   2003
  646.7'0085'2—dc21   2003000082

Printed in the United States of America   8006-7045
Banta, Menasha, WI

10   9   8   7   6   5   4   3   2   1

To Bonnie and David Bennett
whom I have the good fortune to call
Mom and Dad

Contents

Contents

The Really
Busy Woman

When my husband and I are teaching our children to do laundry, we start them out on the towels. Towels are easy to do: they're simple to sort, they don't have to be matched up in pairs, and they have no pockets that might be hiding nasty surprises like ballpoint pens or brown crayons or lip balm, any of which even a perfectly capable, laundry-seasoned adult can accidentally overlook in a wash cycle.

There is, however, one common mistake that my children (and even their father) tend to make with towels. They figure that as long as they can keep smashing those towels into the washing machine, they can keep adding more and more to the load. One day I was working in the kitchen when I heard a horrendous noise emanating from the laundry room in the basement. I rushed down to check it out and found the washer groaning and rocking like a crazed cow. Quickly switching it off, I opened the lid and saw a wad of towels crammed in so tightly I could barely pry them out. Now, I have a large-capacity machine, but it was never meant to hold fourteen, full-size bath towels!

Sure, there were fourteen towels that needed washing that day. But as nice as it would have been to be able to throw them in all at once and get it over with, the washer simply doesn't work that way. All you're doing when you try to stuff that many towels into one load is ruining both the machine and the towels. An overloaded washing machine is thrown out of balance and can't do its job properly.

I understand this principle and have explained it with infinite patience to my husband and to each of my five children in turn. But I still haven't become very adept at applying it in the larger scheme of my life. Believe me—it does apply. I'm always falling prey to the notion that I can get one more thing into the load. This is probably because there is always more to accomplish than I have time or energy to do. I am a fourteen-towel woman stuck in a ten-towel-capacity life. And so I tend to operate frequently on overload.

Almost every woman I know is like this. We are really busy! We overload our days with things that truly need to be done and then drop into bed at night wondering why we feel so out of balance. We need to realize that it's better to have ten clean towels in the morning and four set aside for another day than to have fourteen not-so-clean towels and a broken machine. We're in this life for the long haul—if we don't maintain ourselves properly, we will break down.

There are so many good, worthwhile, important tasks requiring my attention and emotional energy, and yet I have learned that I fritter away a lot of that energy in meaningless, unproductive avenues. This book is my attempt to examine those strength-sapping activities and to figure out how to shake loose of them. It doesn't pretend to address the hard questions of life. We all have tragedies, seasons of trial when we have to reach deep inside for inner resources we may not have even known we had.

Just as often, though, we get mired down not by serious troubles but by the little, gnatlike annoyances that swarm throughout our ordinary days. That's what this book is for: pest control. It's an exercise in clearing away the debris so that we can work on developing those inner resources for when we need them. Mostly, it's an acknowledgment that a lot of what goes wrong, in my life at least, could be alleviated if I would just relax about it!

This is where the chocolate comes in. I adore chocolate. I love it in all its myriad forms—in milkshakes and mousses, in doughnuts and cheesecakes and cream pies, in three-for-a-dollar, grocery-store candy bars and twenty-dollar-a-pound, hand-dipped confections. I buy gourmet hot chocolate mix for myself and big tubs of the bargain kind with those teeny, dried-up marshmallows to decoy the kids away from my stash. They reciprocate on Halloween by tossing me the Mounds and Almond Joys from their bags, hoping to divert me long enough for them to pocket the Snickers and the Peanut M&M's.

Now, I'm not really silly enough to think that chocolate solves anything. But it calms me. It's a soothing assurance that this hectic life I have worked myself into is also full of wonderful surprises and unexpected sweetness. It reminds me that a hefty percentage of my "problems" don't really need to be solved at all, just outlasted.

So here's to chocolate, and to a number of other semi-practical solutions to the woes of everyday life. Whether they help us increase our capacity or diminish our load, there are things we can do to get out of the overload trap we catch ourselves in so often. But when all else fails, bring out the chocolate, and give me—or another close friend—a call if it still hurts in the morning. We're all in this together, after all, and sometimes talking things out is the best solution there could be.

CHAPTER ONE

Know When to Say No

We're not much of a family for airplanes. Our jobs haven't required much flying; we live in the same city as both our extended families; and frankly, with as many kids as we have, it's usually just cheaper to drive on vacations. But one year when we got a larger-than-expected tax refund, we splurged and flew the family to Washington, D.C.

It was a two-legged trip, with a stopover in Chicago, and as we got on the second plane, my husband, Larry, and I found ourselves seated behind the galley. It was kind of nice, actually, with a little extra leg room and no one in front of us leaning their seats back. The disadvantage was that there were no tray tables. Being neophyte fliers, we didn't realize that the trays for those seats were cleverly concealed in the armrests, and no one pointed this out to us. It was a short flight, though, with no meal being served—only drinks and snack mix. We figured it really didn't matter.

Larry settled in with a magazine in his lap, and somehow his snack bag and drink both ended up in his left hand while he was turning pages with his right. This was fine until, without thinking, he went to dump some snack mix directly into his mouth from the bag. I barely caught him out of the corner of my eye just as he poured about six ounces of tomato juice right down the front of his white polo shirt.

Gracious, sympathetic wife that I am, I tried very, very hard not to laugh. I unloaded as much of my mirth as I could while he was in the rest room cubicle trying to sponge himself off. I almost had control of myself as he came out the door, but one look at that shirt just sent me off again. He sat there with a sort of grieved look on his face until I was quite finished, when I apologized and said, "You know, honey, this is going to be funny someday."

"It's funny now," he admitted. "I just don't feel like laughing, is all."

Well, it was funny, and it grows funnier with the retelling and the increased distance from the time of the trauma, but I also think there's a valuable lesson in that experience. We all take on more than we can handle sometimes. Everything seems fine at first, but sooner or later our attention will be diverted, and we'll wind up making a mess of things. It's practically inevitable.

The fact is, we're not so good at saying no. "Will you join

our car pool, our book group, our exercise class, our choir, our lunch bunch?" We're flattered to be asked, and it sounds like so much fun. It's even worse when it comes to our children because we want to be sure they don't miss a single opportunity to develop their talents. We sign right up for piano and ballet and soccer and baseball and Tae Kwon Do and swimming lessons and YMCA arts and crafts class.

When did we lose sight of the fact that saying yes to some things generally implies needing to say no to others? Why does "no" feel like such an admission of defeat? I think for me it's because I'm embarrassed to confess that I simply can't do everything, especially when it seems like every other woman manages to get it all in.

Every other mother is crafting clever Halloween costumes for her children out of common household items while I'm at Wal-Mart digging through the boxes for a size 10 Spiderman suit. Every other woman brings a home-baked masterpiece to the potluck party, while I'm arranging my brownies on a paper plate and trying to ditch the plastic container from the grocery store where I bought them. How can I say no when everyone else is so obviously saying yes? I just need to buck up and do better, I tell myself—get up a little earlier in the morning, be a little more organized, make better lists.

I started thinking a little differently about this one year

over Thanksgiving dinner. My mother-in-law is a fabulous cook on any occasion, but Thanksgiving at her house is truly a remarkable event. For one thing, she has an uncanny knack for remembering what each of her ten children likes most to eat, and she makes certain that everyone's favorites are well represented. Add spouses and grandchildren, and her equal concern for them, and you may get some idea of the spread that fills the kitchen and overflows into the dining room for the grown-ups and the kids' tables in the living room and alcove.

The year I'm speaking of was the year I finally caught on that if you try to eat regular portions of everything that shows up on Thanksgiving in that kitchen, you are going to be sick, sick, sick. It just can't be done. So you have two choices: you can eat a lot of what you like best and skip over the other stuff, or you can take a little taste of everything and get filled up that way. Either alternative seems to work just fine, but if you want to stay well, you do have to choose. Fortunately, however, if you're patient enough to hang around for several hours, you can slip back into the kitchen when you get hungry again and eat something else.

Doesn't it sometimes seem as if life is one giant, all-you-can-eat buffet? And the pain of it is, everything looks good. The trick to not being overcome by all this bounty is to know what you really want, to load up your plate with that, and then to get comfortable with saying no to the rest.

You may have to start with the "little-bit-of-everything" philosophy. Sometimes you just have to do some sampling to see what experiences are worth repeating. This is the driving principle behind most universities' general education programs, which require students to take at least a taste of many different subjects so they can be more well rounded and have a better sense of what would suit them as a lifelong pursuit.

As you go on, though, chances are you'll end up devoting larger chunks of your time to selected responsibilities. I noticed every time we welcomed a child into our family, for instance, that it was like scooping up a huge helping of some really filling dish. For a while, it eclipsed everything else on the plate.

The great thing about having a newborn for me was that it gave me wonderful practice in saying no. (There were other great things about it too, of course, but the "no" thing was a real bonus.) Nurturing a baby utilized every resource I had, physically and mentally and emotionally. I moved in a kind of haze from feeding to feeding, catching a nap when I could and accomplishing only what surface work needed to be done in order to keep the family functioning. I blissfully—and guiltlessly—said no to planning committees and charity drives and room mothering because there was literally no way I could say yes.

No stage in a child's life flies by faster than newborn, though, and it wasn't long before I was anxious to get involved again. This is where it got tricky. A few years ago, I generally had three children attending elementary school in any given year. I couldn't be a room mother for all three! Each year, several organizations would call to ask me to help with their annual fund drives. Honestly, I was hearing from the American Cancer Society, American Heart Association, Primary Children's Medical Center, Multiple Sclerosis Society, March of Dimes—how could I do all of them? But I felt rotten saying no, so I would say yes, and someone would drop off a packet with envelopes and information brochures and donor lists, and I would set it aside until the day before it was due and then spend fifteen grudging, guilt-filled minutes running up and down my street banging on my neighbors' doors. Usually those packets went back with one envelope—mine—containing any kind of donation. Wasn't I a big help? Because I said yes when my heart was screaming no, the work didn't really get done by anybody.

I have a new strategy now. I pick one "cause" a year outside of church and family, and when the others call I tell them, "I'm sorry, I can't be involved this year because I'm focusing my efforts on this other cause." And then I go and do a good job for one group and feel comfortable in that contribution. The world needs volunteers, and we all need meaningful involvement in serving others, but if we're not careful that service will come at the expense of our families, our health, or our sanity.

That sanity is perhaps most threatened, though, not by our own involvement but by that of our children. It can be even harder to say no to worthwhile and fun activities for the kids, probably because we want so much for them to develop their strengths and to feel good about their accomplishments and to find their niche in the world. But it is devilishly easy to overprogram a young child's life, and when multiple children are involved, it can really wreak havoc on a family's unity and stability to be pulled in so many directions. I estimate that I get a flyer sent home from school about every two weeks inviting my children to enroll for some extracurricular sports or drama or music or cheerleading activity. They beg me to sign them up. And I smile and say, "We're doing one music and one other thing this year. Is this the other thing that you choose?" (I chose the music— motherly prerogative!) This helps them discover what they truly want to be involved in, and that way they're more likely to be fully committed to it.

If this seems like too big a change for you all at once, try this idea: drop one thing. Try doing without just one regular activity for yourself or for your children. You might be surprised at how little you miss it, how much you prefer a more relaxed pace and more time to spend together. You can use the time that you saved by saying no to commit yourself more completely to the things you've said yes to. You may discover other things to drop that aren't as vital as you thought.

A word of caution, however: getting into the habit of saying no can be just as dangerous to your well-being as always saying yes. Here are some do's and don'ts you may want to consider.

1. Don't say no to Church callings. If the bishop asks you to accept an assignment, figure out a way that you can say yes to it even if it seems like you can't possibly do it.

Two weeks after I was called as our ward Relief Society president, I found out I was pregnant. I went crying into the bishop's office, and he let me fuss for a while before proposing his solution. "I'll tell you what, Sister Watts," he said. "Let's leave things the way they are for now. But anytime you feel like you might need to be released, you come in here, and you and I will get down on our knees and ask Heavenly Father if it's time to release you, and if he says it is, we'll do it." That was a great lesson to me. The Lord knew I was pregnant when he impressed the bishop to call me to the position. He wasn't asking me to do something I couldn't handle.

Sure enough, I spent nearly three years in that position and never felt inclined to ask for a release, even when we had two funerals a week apart right at Christmastime when I was eight months pregnant. Whom the Lord calls, he magnifies. I found that out.

I'm embarrassed to admit that I have found myself on the other end of the spectrum as far as accepting callings is concerned. One year I was teaching Relief Society, which is really my favorite calling in the Church, and my husband (who was a counselor in the bishopric) asked me to accept a calling as nursery leader. I'll confess it: I was mad. I was in the throes of dealing with nursery-age kids at home; the last thing I wanted to do was mess with them at church as well. I loved my Relief Society assignment and didn't want to give it up. I thought the assignment had been made out of desperation rather than inspiration, and that I had been caught in a trap of, "Sure, my wife will do that." Worst of all, an ugly burst of pride persuaded me that I had "grown beyond" that kind of calling.

I tried to turn it down, but my husband was persistent. He invited me to go home and pray about it. Wouldn't you know it, I felt almost instantly a loving rebuke that seemed to say, Can't you do this little thing for me? I went back and accepted the call, and though I started it with a grudging heart, I soon began to truly enjoy it. There were little blessings waiting for me around almost every corner in that season, and I would have deprived myself of all of them if I hadn't said yes even though it was hard to make myself do it.

2. Do be willing to sacrifice something you want to do if there's something else you need to be involved in that is more important. For years I have enjoyed singing in a local chorus. One year the regular weekly rehearsal night conflicted with our ward's Young Women activity night, and I was serving in the presidency of that organization. I thought I had done a long enough "stint," so I asked the bishop to release me so I wouldn't have to quit the choir. It wasn't very many weeks before I knew in my heart that I had chosen wrong. It was almost impossible for me to enjoy participating in the choir that year because I constantly felt that it wasn't where I was supposed to be at that time in my life.

After that experience, I vowed that if I ever felt again that there was something that I needed to be doing, even if it meant giving up the chorus, I would do it. Sure enough, I have had the opportunity to test that resolve twice more since then. Both times, although I thought it would break my heart, I took an extended leave of absence from the choir. And both times the choice has brought me peace and

I have been able to accomplish what I felt was truly necessary without feeling deprived, even though I had given up something I loved. I'll always be grateful for the seasons in my life when I was able to be fully committed to the chorus and to enjoy the learning and the satisfaction of singing the world's great music. But I'm equally grateful for the other avenues I've been free to explore because I was willing to set that aside for a time.

3. Don't let yourself become a martyr by always being the one to make the sacrifice. Going back to the years I did sing in the chorus, I can point out dozens of sacrifices my family made in order for me to do so. It didn't hurt them too much to find out that Mom was a real person, with needs and talents and responsibilities that didn't all revolve around them.

I've found the same to be true at work. Just about any job worth giving your heart to will take every ounce of time and attention you're willing to spend on it. If you're always the one who takes on one more project and ends up staying two hours later at night or slipping in on Saturdays, you may be digging a hole for yourself that will be hard to climb out of one day. Sometimes work comes first, but other times your family will take precedence, or church, or service, or friends. Be sure you get your own needs to the top of the to-do list once in a while, too.

4. Do take heart from the fact that things change. You may feel completely buried for a while under a toddler's demands or a huge work deadline or a complicated project you've taken on at home. It's hard to imagine you'll ever feel normal again. The stress of it follows you to bed at night and washes over you the moment you awake in the morning.

Take a deep breath and keep pressing forward. Toddlers grow. Deadlines pass. Projects get done. You'll get your life back before you know it—and then you'll turn around and give it to some other pursuit. If you've learned to say no to things that don't matter, the times you say yes will be filled with joy and growth and, most of all, peace.

CHAPTER TWO

Negotiate a Lasting Peace with Your Body

Anyone who thinks that stress is all in a person's mind has no concept of how much of it I carry around my waistline. The fact is, stress is clearly a complex interplay between mind and body. I have seen how big a role my body plays in my own emotional state.

Until I got to junior high, I was on pretty good terms with my body. Sure, we had the occasional tiff about its being too slow or too awkward—but not until my early teens did I start seeing my body as my enemy. For one thing, those are the years when the body unleashes the biological weapons we know as hormones, so everything is out of control for a couple of years anyway. Lump together in one classroom a bunch of kids who are feeling especially insecure about themselves and don't have the life experience to channel that insecurity appropriately, and you're looking for trouble.

Of all the classes in junior high that contributed to these feelings of inadequacy, gym, or phys. ed., as we called it in the 1960s, topped the list. In my junior high days, there was no such thing as coed gym class. There was a girls' gymnasium and a boys', with a fold-up wall between them that could be moved for varsity basketball games. We girls all wore the standard-issue uniform: a royal blue, one-piece jumpsuit with short, cuffed sleeves and legs about to the knee, plus white sneakers with our names printed along the side with a black marker. Changing into that gym suit in an open room in full view of forty or fifty other girls was the first horror.

It paled in comparison, though, with Friday afternoons in the wintertime, when we abandoned our normal routine to undertake a course in ballroom dancing. The barrier between the two gymnasiums came down, and the gym coaches, who were all clearly more comfortable with a basketball in their hands, attempted to guide us through the finer points of the waltz and the cha-cha. On Fridays we didn't have to wear the gym suits. We stayed in our dresses (no pants for girls in school back then) and just changed into our gym shoes so as not to scuff the floor.

Of course, the most difficult thing about teaching a bunch of ninth-graders to dance is pairing them off. The teachers had several inventive ways of doing this, but the one I remember best is where they had all the girls line up against one wall of the gym, facing the wall, and the boys line up at the opposite wall. Then, at the blast of the coach's whistle, the boys were to walk across the room to tap the girl of their choice on the shoulder and politely ask, "May I have this dance?"

Reasonable in theory. Miserable in practice. There is no experience that quite compares with standing with your nose to the wall, listening to a thundering horde of footsteps (the supposed walk across the room was always more like a stampede) and knowing that none of them are coming in your direction. Like huge electromagnets gathering up straight pins, the four or five most popular girls would suck all the traffic their way, leaving us geeks on the periphery to anguish for two or three long, increasingly quiet minutes until we finally felt the tap and heard the resigned query, "Wanna dance?" Or, worse, on some days there would be another whistle blast and a cruel announcement: "Okay, there are no more boys left, so the rest of you girls, partner up with each other." I, having attained my full six-foot stature by then, was frequently left to play the boy's part. I got so adept at leading, in fact, that once when I was in college actually dancing with a real boy, I anticipated one of his leads incorrectly and dealt him a right cross that bloodied his lip.

In short, ninth-grade dance class was about as much fun as boot camp. It seemed to have a similar effect of tearing down one's self-esteem, but without the corresponding compensation of rebuilding the individual as part of a unit filled with *esprit de corps*. In junior high it was every woman for herself, and my self took a rather a serious emotional battering.

I'm not blaming the boys at my junior high for all this pain, you understand. At that point in time, six feet was not yet recognized as the height to which supermodels would one day aspire. I was a full head taller than most ninth-graders, and it was as awkward for me as it was for the boy to try to waltz with his head right at the level . . . well, suffice it to say it was just as well that I didn't have much of a figure. I'm not looking for sympathy, though—I tell this miserable story only to explain how it was that I began to be at war with my body.

Another junior high experience was less the fault of my body than of my ego, but it was still another log on the hating-my-body fire. This time the class was home economics, and we were doing a sewing unit, making a simple jumper. When it came time to select our patterns, I was too embarrassed to admit that my measurements dictated the purchase of a girls' size 12. I fudged by a couple of inches to land in the "Young Junior Teen" category.

After a semester of agony, with more unpicking and restitching and downright weeping than I care to remember, I put on the almost-finished jumper (I had to tape the hem up with masking tape because I ran out of time) to wear in the class fashion show. I strolled down the makeshift runway between the desks, did the obligatory twirl at the end, and waited for the teacher's evaluation. "A nice effort," she pronounced, "but the darts are a little too big." This elicited a round of snickers from my peers, and I'm sure I blushed beet-red as I hurried back down the runway, tears stinging my eyes.

Although it wasn't a conscious choice, I believe I concluded through my accumulated humiliations in junior high that I couldn't be pretty, that I would never be pretty, and that therefore I would never make any real attempt to fix myself up physically. Today, with decades of hindsight guiding me, I can see how wrong that was. True, I was six feet tall, and nothing I could do was ever going to change that. But I had good hair, and clear skin, and I was thin and even sort of good at a few sports, like basketball and tennis.

However, I was at war with my body, and that meant I would not treat it well. I didn't keep it very clean or feed it with the best sorts of food or attempt to clothe it nicely. My "I-don't-care" attitude virtually guaranteed that I would not feel good about the way I looked. I'm ashamed to admit that

I even became a little contemptuous of girls who did spend time and money on their appearance, branding such behavior as "shallow" and considering myself "above all that."

This attitude followed me into adulthood, wreaking more havoc than I care to acknowledge. I had developed horrendous eating habits in my teenage years, and they really sabotaged me once I hit about age thirty and my metabolism slowed way down. I hated clothes shopping with a passion, because a three-way mirror destroyed the illusion I still harbored of myself as a thin woman. I often put off buying new clothes, especially pants, thinking I would just "lose ten pounds" and then come back and try them. I guess I've been trying to "lose ten pounds" for about twenty-five years. Obviously, one can't put off buying new clothes for a quarter century, so for years I bought the cheapest things I could find, believing somehow that I didn't deserve nice clothes and wouldn't invest in them until I had the figure I really wanted.

I hit a low point in all this mess the day my fourth child was born. It was the first time I had had an epidural block for a childbirth, and one of my early thoughts after the excitement of the delivery had died down was that I wanted to pound anyone who had ever tried to talk me out of that anesthesia. I know, I know, it's not right for everyone, but I've got to tell you, it was like heaven to me. I felt great! I made all the calls myself to tell our family we had a new baby brother. I loved everything about it.

Except one thing. The epidural numbs all the feeling in your lower body, which means that you can't move your legs until it wears off. So when it was time to shift me from the delivery bed to my hospital bed so they could wheel me off to the maternity ward, the nurses were on their own. My legs lay helpless on the sheet, like twin beached dolphins, and when the poor little nurse tried to heft one of them over onto the other bed, she had a terrible time of it. I don't know how much one of my legs weighs when it's truly dead weight, but apparently it's more than one nurse can handle. She had to summon in a whole backup squad to hoist me over. It was, to put it mildly, an embarrassing moment.

I brooded about this for a while, but the sad truth is that when I brood, I eat, so things didn't get any better at that point. I went through a several-year period of waving off well-meaning, solicitous people, apparently eager to share in my joy, who assumed I was pregnant and asked when my baby was due. One time the clerk at the grocery store handed me a strip of stickers, saying, "For the little one," and I didn't have any "little ones" with me. I suppose it would have been a really sweet and clever gesture if I *had* been pregnant, but it fell rather short considering that my youngest child was eight. However, it's easier just to smile and take the stickers than to try to explain, so that's what I did. Then I went home and started thinking about that phenomenon and what it was doing to my life. The inner dialogue went something like this:

"Are you going to try to lose some weight or aren't you?"

"Probably someday. But not now."

"Why not?"

"Dieting takes up a huge chunk of emotional energy. It's more than I've got to give right now."

"So, you're not going to diet right now."

"Correct."

"Because it takes too much emotional energy."

"Yes."

"So why are you spending all this emotional energy bemoaning the fact that your body looks the way it does, when you have no intention of doing anything at the moment about the way your body looks?"

I had me there!

This was a revelation of sorts to me that I was caught in a nasty cycle of negativity that was only making my problems worse. I decided at that moment that it was time to call a truce with my body. Although I wasn't ready to diet, I thought there might be other things I could do to feel better about myself and at least slow down the emotional downhill slide I seemed to be trapped on.

I started by making a list of all the wonderful things my body could do. I was truly amazed to contemplate the blessing of good health I had enjoyed for most of my life. I began to appreciate my body as the vehicle for all the things I loved to do: my eyes, which could read and watch my children play and drink in the beauty of a spring day; my ears, which could hear music and laughter and cheerful conversation; my arms and hands, which could lift an infant and fix a meal and throw a Frisbee; and even my twin-dolphin legs, which could usually get me where I wanted to go if I didn't expect them to run for long stretches. It came to me gradually: My body was not my enemy! It was not something to fear, to hold an uneasy truce with—a truce I was bound to break the terms of every time I wanted a bite of chocolate.

My body was my ally, my great friend in the adventure we call mortality, one of the reasons for my having come to this life in the first place. I could love it, even in its flawed, less-than-perfect, un-model-like state. I could do the best I could with the body I had, and see where that took me.

This may seem like a silly jumping-off point to some, but the first thing I did was to buy some really lovely scented lotion for my dry skin. Rubbing that lotion in was an exercise in spending time with my long-neglected body. Of course, when my children observed that it smelled like I was massaging my heels with Kool-Aid, it put a bit of a damper on things, but I found I preferred the fruits to the florals in the lotion department, and this was *my* indulgence, after all, so I just ignored my detractors and pressed on.

Next I got a haircut. This was a huge step for a woman who had worn her hair long and straight for a couple of decades, and it took me quite a while to get comfortable with the idea. I experimented over the months with different lengths until I hit on a look that I liked and could re-create even with my limited cosmetological skill.

Clothes were the hardest part. There aren't a lot of choices for a woman who is both big and tall, but I was determined to get out of the loose, flowing dresses that were so easily mistaken for maternity outfits. I was absorbed in watching *The X-Files* at the time, and when I realized that the main character was pregnant in real life and they were trying to disguise it for as long as they could on the show, I started paying close attention to what she wore. Jackets. Open sweaters. Longer skirts. I started adding pieces to my wardrobe, and the questions about my pending pregnancy dwindled to nothing.

For years I avoided getting a makeover, on the grounds that if someone did doll me all up, and I still didn't like the way I looked, I would have dashed all hopes that I *could* look better if I wanted to expend the effort. But one day I had to appear on a videotape for work, and I knew one couldn't do that sort of thing bare-faced, so I marched in and put myself in the hands of the ladies at the cosmetic counter. They worked me over pretty seriously, and I was grateful for it, but it was clearly never going to be my style. I do wear a little makeup—blush and eye shadow and, for special occasions, lipstick—but I don't think it's ever going to be very important to me.

I'm still working on my eating habits. I haven't gotten to the point of dieting yet, but I am trying to treat myself to more healthy foods and to get up from my desk and walk around more often. My weight hovers within about a five-pound radius, and when my pants get too tight I lay off the Peanut M&M's for a couple of weeks to swing myself down to the lower end of that range.

Most of all, just as I have always wanted people to love me for who I am, and not the way I look, I'm learning to love my body for what it can do, not just the way it looks. All the most important things about it have less to do with its appearance than with its functionality, and I am thankful every day of my life to be able to get up out of my bed and go to work and take care of my family and enjoy my life. The tremendous stress of being at war with my body has disappeared. Sure, I hope to continue improving and moving forward, getting in better shape and operating well for as long as possible, but in the meantime I can say that I'm truly at peace.

What would it take for you to be friends with your body? Try starting today with a "thankful list" of every blessing your body has given you access to, and see if it doesn't make a difference in how you look at things. You'll be amazed at how much stress disappears when you and your body are working on the same side!

CHAPTER THREE

Quit Trying to Finish the Laundry

I wonder if there lurks deep within the heart of every woman a secret, irrational belief that if she could just once finish every bit of laundry in the house, she would achieve some Nirvana-like higher plane of housekeeping consciousness. It's as if we think there's a Laundry Fairy out there who will touch us on the head with her wand and decree that we'll never have to do laundry again—if we can just get it *all* done one time.

This is a fool's hope, because unless you strip every member of your family naked for at least the amount of time it takes to run a wash-and-dry cycle, they are generating new laundry even as you're tossing the last sock from the hamper into the washing machine. And even if you do get every last one of those socks washed, the chances of them all coming out of the dryer with their mates intact are approximately one in seven million. I actually dreamed once that we were moving from our house, and when we hauled the washer and dryer out of the basement we found under and behind them all the socks we had lost over the years.

I finally gave up trying to win the hosiery war and began buying socks for my three boys in packages of several dozen identical pairs. Then I still had trouble matching them because the boys seemed to dirty them at different rates, and I couldn't bring myself to fold a nice, white sock together with one that was permanently gray along the sole of the foot. I make them match their own socks now because it's just too depressing to me.

Face it—the laundry is never going to be done. And it's not just the laundry. No matter how sumptuously you fed your family today, chances are they're going to want to eat again tomorrow. The meticulously trimmed lawn will be shaggy in a couple of weeks. The dog will need walking, the floor will need mopping, the furniture will need dusting, the sink will need scrubbing, and Old Man River, he jes' keeps rollin' along.

Most of us live in denial of the fact that so many of the tasks of our lives partake of this cyclical, unfinished nature. We like closure. We like to finish things. And so we live in mild despair, feeling as though we're never accomplishing anything because nothing seems to *stay* accomplished.

We clearly need a new way of looking at this issue. I, for

one, do not propose to let my life slip past me unnoticed because I'm too preoccupied holding my husband's socks up to the light to distinguish the black ones from the navy blue. But what can be done?

My fifth-grade son devised one solution that worked well for him until I found out about it. He sleeps in the basement, where it gets pretty cold, and he came up one evening displaying his nightwear, which he called his "ACCC," or Anti-Coldness Containment Center. It consisted of sweats, top and bottom, and a couple of extra shirts underneath. He liked to have names and sound effects for his self-constructed reality, and hey, if he was happy, I was happy.

I'm not terribly observant, especially in the mornings when the kids are rushing to get off to school and I'm trying to get ready for work. But it finally clicked in my brain one day that this child had worn the same shirt out the door several days running. Upon investigation, I found out that what he was doing was putting the ACCC on *over* his clothing so he wouldn't have to go to the bother of getting undressed every night and then dressed again the next morning. Although this is admittedly a creative solution for dealing with the monotony of repetitious tasks, it's not an acceptable one, even for an eleven-year-old boy. So we need to look elsewhere for answers.

I think the first step we need to take is to let go of our

denial and accept the fact that as long as we're alive and kicking, there are going to be some jobs that will have to be done again and again. Knowing that this is the way the world works, we can then set about asking ourselves what we can gain from it.

One immediately evident benefit of the phenomenon of never-finished business is that it teaches us to value process over product. Since "products" seem to be few and far between, whereas "process" is with us every day, it makes sense that we'll be happier if we can learn to relax and enjoy *doing* as much as we enjoy *finishing*.

"Are we there yet? Are we there yet?" It's not a phrase you hear when you're sitting in the little boat at Disneyland moving through "Pirates of the Caribbean." Everyone knows that you stand in line for the ride, not for the turnstile that signals its end. What if we treated life the same way?

Often, tasks that need to be done over and over again bring order to the chaos of our lives. The law of entropy suggests that a thing left to itself will decay over time. This is certainly true of my living room! Restoring order when things are in disarray can be a very soothing activity.

Once when our family was on vacation, racing from museums to historic sites to monuments, we took some time one evening to do some grocery shopping. The sense of normalcy involved in picking out good apples and checking the eggs in the carton and verifying the freshness date on the milk brought an immediate feeling of calm over the frenetic mood that had prevailed that day.

Something about the repetition of our ordinary jobs creates a rhythm that engages us in our lives on a daily basis. It's instructive to me that the Lord's Prayer includes the line, "Give us this day our daily bread." It brings to mind the Israelites gathering manna, which they had to do every day except the Sabbath. Why? God obviously could have sent it to them each week instead of every day; wouldn't that have been less monotonous, a more efficient use of their time? But he purposely made it so they couldn't gather and hoard extra even if they tried. What is there about the notion of "daily bread" that serves his purposes?

I wonder if he wanted the Israelites to have faith, every single day of their lives, that he was going to sustain them for one more day. I wonder if he wants us to know, every day of our lives, that he will help us do the things that are most important for us to do, that the time we are given will be sufficient for the day, and that we'll get a whole new, fresh supply of hours tomorrow. I wonder if he is actually giving us the opportunity, every single day, to rediscover the greatest blessings of our lives.

Think about this for a minute. I could go to the grocery store tomorrow, buy a bag of apples and a loaf of bread and a jar of peanut butter, and eat better all week than many people eat in their lives. I wouldn't have to cook, and I wouldn't have to do any dishes. I could eliminate those mundane tasks just like that! Similarly, I could wear the same dress to work every day, with a special second outfit reserved for Sundays, as I'm sure my foremothers did. That would cut down on my laundry considerably.

But I don't want to live that way. I like having lots of choices in clothing to suit my moods. I love eating a variety of foods. The fact that such abundance is available to me is something to celebrate! Cooking and cleaning and laundry are simply the foundation stones that support the enormous pile of blessings that my family enjoys.

Of course, sometimes those foundation stones seem like rocks piling on top of me until I can hardly breathe. It helps at such times to remember that, since I will never be *ultimately* finished with these tasks until I die, I need to allow myself to be *temporarily* finished with them on a regular basis.

One of my favorite television shows from my childhood was *The Flintstones*. Do you remember how each episode began? A loud, train-type whistle signaled the end of Fred's workday, and he slid down the back of his brontosaurus shouting "Yabba-dabba-doo!" Sure, he would be back at work tomorrow, but for a while he was finished with the rock pit and could do what he chose.

Try blowing the whistle on your workday at a certain point each day—a point that leaves you some time and energy to do what *you* choose. Say to yourself, "I'm off the clock now," and don't punch back in until the next day, no matter how many chores seem to scream for your attention. Know that you'll get to them all in good time, and when you do, they'll go much more smoothly and seem less irksome because you're coming to them fresh.

Then give yourself some points for what you accomplished today. Did the children all go to school with clean socks? Ten points for you! Take another five for running the dishwasher and actually getting it emptied, ten for vacuuming the living room, and twenty if you fixed a nutritious dinner (boxed mixes count). Score five points for every phone call you fielded at work, with a bonus five if the person was a grump. Ten points for a piece of paper gone from your desk for good. You'll be surprised how these points add up! You're accomplishing much more than you realize.

The labors we're talking about here have a tendency to be tedious, so anything you can do to make them less tiresome works in your favor. I, for one, am grateful to live in an age when so many things are automated. The direct deposit option for our paychecks saves me all kinds of time at the bank—not to mention its eliminating the embarrassment I used to experience if I didn't get there quite soon enough to make that deposit. One of my happier days in life was the day workmen finished putting in our automatic sprinklers, signaling the end of my lugging around a little sprinkler head at the end of a hose to place it at a different spot on the lawn every half hour for a day and a half, three times a week. And when my daughter wanted to play the flute in the school band, I remembered our earlier experience renting her brother's violin, which may have placed our credit rating in jeopardy because I was always forgetting to send in the payment. I signed right up on the dotted line to have the flute rental charge deducted automatically from our credit card account. If a thing can do itself, I say, let it do so!

For those things that require hands-on involvement, though, treat yourself to the right tools for the job whenever you can. When I lived in an apartment with friends before my marriage, we had a vacuum that we pretty much had to hand feed. Sometimes, if you picked up a scrap of something and tossed it into the middle of the room where you could run over it five or six times, it would get sucked in, but it was easier just to detach the wand, crawl around and pick up the bits of debris with your fingers, and shove them directly into the nozzle. Needless to say, we were not frequent vacuumers.

I'm all for labor-saving devices, if you can afford them and have room for them, and if they're saving you labor on things you do regularly. I once had a deluxe mixer on a stand that came with a bread hook and other exotic attachments, but it was hard to store and hard to dig out of the cupboard, and I rarely made bread anyway. I gave it up for a good, sturdy hand mixer that slips easily into a drawer, and *that* is an appliance that I use several times a week. I also plunked down the money for a really solid wire whisk, a decent set of measuring spoons, and a great potato peeler, and it's astonishing how much less annoying the tasks related to those items have become.

Another way to beat tedium in the kitchen is to try new recipes. We have a peanut butter escape clause at our house so that if the kids really can't gag down what I fixed for dinner they can make their own sandwiches. This leaves me free to experiment with different dishes every once in a while. We also have a code phrase that conveys gently a person's opinion that a given experiment ought not to be repeated: "Well, that was nice to try once." This acknowledges the good intentions of the cook and encourages the trying of new things while not dooming the family to repeated endurings of a yucky entrée.

Don't hesitate to share the blessings of repetitive work. It's just more fun for children to roll up socks if they're racing against the champion. And somehow I don't mind scrubbing the tub so much if my husband is cheerfully wiping down the walls in the hall. I feel a lot less resentful and less put upon when the whole family or the roommates are all working together for the common good. It seems to validate the labor somehow, which is crucial for tasks that are likely to feel undone again almost the moment that you complete them.

Another useful trick is to finish, every now and then, some job that will *stay* finished, at least for a good, long while. Paint a room. Create a scrapbook page. Learn a new piece on the piano. Frame a picture. Take a bag of used clothing to Deseret Industries or the Salvation Army—that's twenty-five pounds of stuff you'll never have to look at again. These little islands of accomplishment in a sea of unfinished business can be welcome resting places for your psyche.

If things have just built up to a point where you want to take a match to the whole pile, call a time-out from the usual chores of the day and take a few hours to get yourself back to ground level, at least in some areas. My husband, who is one of ten children, says that once a year or so, his parents would just gather up every scrap of clothing that had accumulated in the laundry room and the kids' bedrooms, and head over to the Laundromat where they could wash it all at once.

I get this way at work sometimes, especially when things get hectic or I find myself in a lot of meetings. Piles of papers stack up on my desk and credenza, quietly reproducing (I'm convinced of this) while they're waiting to be filed or acted upon or decided about. When it gets to the point that I can't even determine what to work on next, and my brain is in a blur of despair over what needs to be accomplished, I set everything aside and start going systematically through the stacks. My office chair, which sits on wheels, usually ends up doing duty as a hand truck for the piles of paper on their way to the recycle bin down the hall. I may not have gotten a thing done that day, but I've paved the way to get twice as much done each day for the rest of the week.

The stacks will be back. I'm resigned to that. Sometimes, though, we do move to a higher level of understanding or commitment that allows us to do those things in a different way. For example, I don't expect I'll ever be able to shut my scriptures and say, "Well, that's it. I get Isaiah at last. I don't have to read that book ever again." I will always need to read my scriptures, because they will say different things to me each time I read them. I don't even have to switch translations!

Take Isaiah. After having participated in a local "*Messiah*

Sing-In" for many Christmas seasons, I was slogging through the Isaiah passages in Second Nephi when I happened upon this verse: "For unto us a child is born, unto us a son is given; and the government shall be upon his shoulder; and his name shall be called, Wonderful, Counselor, The Mighty God, The Everlasting Father, The Prince of Peace" (2 Nephi 19:6; see also Isaiah 9:6). I stopped in amazement. I thought, "This is in *Isaiah?* But I get this! I understand this verse!" It sort of made up for all the stuff in the first verse of that chapter about Zebulun and Naphtali that I wasn't quite grasping. It gave me hope that there might be other verses in this section that would have meaning for me—and indeed there were, and will continue to be more and more, I hope, as I get better and better at deciphering them.

So I'll keep reading. And I'll keep washing clothes, and fixing meals, and answering phones, and doing all the things that make up the fabric of my life, and one day I'll present the whole cloth to my Father in heaven and hope that he judges my work worthy of his kingdom. Meanwhile, I'll relax and enjoy the weaving!

CHAPTER FOUR

Recapture Some Pea-Shelling Time

I f there were a receiving line somewhere in heaven to admit us into the presence of the people who invented things like the washing machine, the microwave oven, and the refrigerator, I would be the first person to stand in it. I am so grateful not to live in pioneer times, I could weep. I observed to my mother once, when we were hiking as a family and I was huffing and puffing, that I would have been a real hindrance to a handcart company. "No, you wouldn't, sweetheart," she assured me, "you'd get whipped into shape in no time." Then, glancing at me with a grin, she added, "That, or you'd collapse on the second day and they would bury you beside the trail. Either way, you wouldn't slow them down any."

Be that as it may, I am unabashed in my gratitude for modern conveniences.

I recently attended a Relief Society fall social in a ward

where many of the women were in their seventies and eight-ies. The committee was running a little behind, and as they were rushing about to finish setting the tables, someone remarked, "It's a lucky thing Sister Somebody isn't here to see this." My friend who had invited me to the party explained that when Sister Somebody had been Relief Society president years earlier, she had insisted that the peas for dinner be hand-shelled. I looked around at the forty or so women who had arrived already and wondered how long it would take to shell peas for a group that size. Sending up a silent prayer of thanks for my freezer at home, I made some comment about how times had changed. One of the sisters agreed, "Oh, I know. They used to have to sit here all afternoon just to get the peas ready. Can you imagine?"

Well, I could imagine, and I did. The funny thing was, when I imagined it, the thought of a bunch of women sitting in a circle talking and laughing as they shelled peas together was actually kind of an attractive one. I felt a little wistful that I had never had that experience. I'm not saying I want to go out and hand-shell my family's peas for the rest of my life, but I do have to admit that in the middle of all we have gained from our time-and-labor-saving miracle appliances, there are a few things we have given up. We as women are not as connected as we used to be.

I had an experience that helped me understand a little

better why this is so. My husband had telephoned me, excited over a kitchen cupboard he had found at a scratch-and-dent sale in the parking lot of a major furniture store. I jumped right in the car, drove out to meet him, and found him hovering protectively over a little corner unit that was perfect for our kitchen. He showed me where the wood in the back had been cracked in one spot, but demonstrated how easy it would be to fix that. We got the piece for a song and drove home exulting in our good fortune.

After rather a lot of gentle reminding and finally outright nagging on my part, my husband got out the carpenter's glue and the C-clamps and joined up the broken wood. Whenever he does a job like this, he likes to call the children around so they can learn from it, and I heard him explaining how important it was that the wood not be moved for several hours, or until the glue was truly dry. "It may seem dry enough in an hour or so," he said, "but it takes longer for a solid bond to form."

That phrase really struck me: It takes time to form lasting bonds. That's true of glued-together items, and it's true of relationships. As the pace of our lives increases, we're less apt to spend the time with each other that brings us together in solid friendship. It's quite a paradox, that we've saved all this time with our modern conveniences and yet find ourselves busier than ever. Our work as women used to bring us together naturally. We need to pay more conscious attention to finding ways for our leisure to do the same thing.

Fortunately, as busy as we are, we all need to stop and eat sometime. This provides a natural opportunity to get together. How hard is it to pick up the phone and invite a friend to meet you for lunch? And Larry and I have rarely had another couple say no to a dinner invitation. There is, however, a trick to this.

You have to be willing to be the one to make the call. Every time, if necessary. If you want to stay connected, take responsibility for the connection.

This is not a dating relationship, after all. You're not testing the waters to see who likes the other one the best. We've found that many of the people we know and love are as busy as we are, and they love to get together but just never seem to get around to calling. We're happy to be the ones to set things up, and when we do connect with these people, even if it has been months since we've seen each other, it's as if we never parted. These are the friendships worth cultivating— any effort we have to put forth is well repaid in the support and love and understanding we reap in return.

When I was home with small children all day, there were times when I thought I would go crazy from the isolation. I swear there were some days I could actually feel my brain sloshing around in my skull, getting softer and mushier from lack of normal adult conversation. I knew enough from talking to women at church that I was not the only one who felt this way, but five minutes of conversation once a week after a three-hour block of meetings with two preschoolers plucking at my pantyhose was hardly sufficient to fill that void in my life.

I finally figured out that if I was ever going to get together with these women the way I wanted to, I had to make it easy for all of us. I called four of them and offered this plan: Wednesday at noon was lunch day at my house. Everyone brought lunch for herself and her kids, and the little ones would go downstairs to play in the basement while the moms talked upstairs. No one needed to feel obligated to come every time, and you didn't have to RSVP or worry about checking in. We kept it really loose, and it was a welcome break in the week and a good incentive for me to keep my living room cleaned up.

A similar plan was explained to me by a friend who had been involved in a monthly study group for several years. They had a rule that the only refreshment ever served when they got together was ice water. This relieved them of the burden of preparing and cleaning up, and allowed them to focus on the purpose of the meeting, which was the material they were studying. Except for a once-a-year

Christmastime potluck, they followed this rule, and I'm sure it helped keep their group running.

Connecting with friends doesn't have to be complicated or expensive. The ease of e-mail helps us stay close to a lot of people we rarely get to see. Then when we do get together, we don't feel like strangers. We're also big proponents of group friendships. If you're lucky enough to know a family or two with kids close to your children's ages, invite them to meet you at the park for a game of Frisbee or tag or soccer. If you have a group of girlfriends at work, drag them out to the food court in the mall once in a while for lunch. Better yet, drag them to your car and get away to some less familiar venue sometimes. Always have a couple of places in mind, so you don't get caught in the old cycle of, "What do you want to do?" "I dunno, what do you feel like?"

One great point of connection is the shared project. One year, two friends of mine got me involved in a Christmas craft that turned into a huge assembly line of stitching, stuffing, and assembling. It was a lot of fun, we spent many great hours together, and I got help making hand-crafted gifts for my family that I wouldn't have been smart enough to make on my own.

Stop right now and think of at least one person you haven't seen for a while whom you'd love to visit with. Pick up the phone, make the call, and enjoy the blessing of being connected. Create your own pea-shelling time!

The other side of shelling peas and making connections that we seem to have lost in the hurry of our present world is a more personal one. I got thinking about this one Christmas when I was dipping cashews. This is a treat my great-aunt used to make, and it's very simple—you just melt white chocolate and then hold a whole cashew by its "tail," dip the wide part into the chocolate, and set it on a piece of waxed paper to dry. These look and taste elegant but can be made by even the homemaking-impaired woman, which of course makes them entirely suitable to my purposes.

Anyway, dipping cashews is similar to shelling peas in many respects: it is somewhat labor intensive but doesn't require a lot of thought once you get into the rhythm of it. And in spite of the fact that I'm running around like an over-wound toy trying to get things ready for Christmas every year, I always take time to dip some cashews. It just seems to calm me down, to set the stage for a happier season, to untangle the mess in my mind.

It occurred to me one year as I was settling in with a batch of nuts and chocolate that we don't have the "thinking time" we used to as women. Our household tasks have become so technology driven that they're finished in practically no time, leaving us free to hurry off to the next chore.

This is great, but the downside is that we just keep piling things up in our minds and don't ever get the time to sort through them. This can cause a tremendous amount of stress.

Have you ever had something come up that you just didn't have time to deal with at the moment, so you set it aside in your brain to think about later? That's what I'm talking about. The more I hurry through a day, the more to-dos of that sort present themselves, and I keep packing them in and hoping for a leisure moment to resolve them. If I don't get time to stop and think, though, they rattle around in my brain unrestricted, and every time one of them surfaces I get more and more panicked because I haven't taken care of it yet.

It's like my e-mail at work. When I get a message in my In Box, I usually read it right away so I can respond immediately if I need to. If the message contains information that I'm going to need later or requires action that I'm not in a position to take right then, I keep the letter in my In Box so I'll remember that I need to get back to it. This system works pretty well most of the time, but now and then I get so busy that I don't take time to sort through those e-mails. To my increasing horror, they start mounting up, until I have three or four hundred messages that I have not yet resolved what to do with. Many of them will have become obsolete and can be deleted easily. There are always a few, though, that cause my stomach to lurch when I realize I haven't done anything about them yet. Talk about stress! I'm a lot more at ease when I'm on top of the In Box pile.

My mind is like a big In Box where I store the ideas and concerns that I still need to work through in some way. When I'm doing a repetitive task, like dipping cashews, I find that I can take these thoughts one at a time and examine them more logically. Many of them get resolved or just disappear altogether when I have time to ponder. But I can't be sitting and dipping cashews every day; I have to look for other ways to build quiet thinking time into my routine.

When our oldest daughter was in high school, she found a special place up in a nearby canyon where she would go when she needed to sort out her life. She called it her "thinking rock," and she found a lot of peace and answers in the solitude there. Having a dedicated spot like that can serve as a trigger to open your heart and mind more effectively. Any quiet corner will do.

I hadn't realized, until I examined my habits more closely, how much of my life I fill with noise. If I do happen to come home to a quiet house—a rarity, I'll admit—I almost instinctively go in and flip on the TV. I tell myself I'm doing this to "unwind," but the truth is that the television doesn't do anything to sort out the jumble of my thoughts. All it really does is shut the thinking part of my brain off. This may help me escape for a little while, but it doesn't give me any lasting help. I can tell this is true because I've noticed I'm more tired and grumpy when I come home from work exhausted and spend an evening watching TV than I am when I come home tired but have another obligation and have to keep moving in the evening.

One of the smarter things I've done has been to make my car a place of refuge. Instead of resenting the time I spend commuting, I have come to relish it. I sing at the top of my voice, I pray, and I hold long conversations with myself in which I plan my days. I know that sounds kind of ridiculous, but you wouldn't believe how effective it can be to verbalize your concerns, even if the person you're telling them to is yourself.

I know people who get up to meditate early in the morning, people who take long walks in the evening, and people who disappear during their lunch hour to someplace quiet. Some people sort things out while they're exercising; others sit quietly with music in the background and run through deep-breathing techniques. There are lots of possibilities—the important thing is to find something that reconnects you with your core being and helps restore your sense of balance and peace. If all else fails, find some peas to shell!

CHAPTER FIVE

Empty Your Recycle Bin

I remember the first time I tried to delete a file from our computer. It was a lot of years ago, but the reason I remember it is because I thought the little message that came up in the pop-up window was so cute: "Are you sure you want to send File X to the Recycle Bin?" It cracked me up that they had built in a feature called a "Recycle Bin." Why not just delete the file when asked?

A month or two later, I found out why not. I had accidentally deleted a file that I still needed, and I was moaning and groaning about it when one of my kids came down and said, with that "duh" in his voice, "Mom, just take it out of the Recycle Bin." I found out then that the Recycle Bin was a repository for things you meant to delete but might want to have another look at before doing so. Ultimately, when you're truly sure you can safely get rid of those files, you can push another button called "Empty Recycle Bin" and have them disappear altogether.

This seems like a good idea for a computer. In real life, however, I think maybe it's not so great. I find that a lot of stress builds up around things that I meant to let go of and haven't quite been able to. This includes both physical junk and emotional traumas. The physical stuff has become easier: I just take a deep breath and shove it in a black plastic sack that I can't see through (so I can't second-guess myself), and I haul it away before I can change my mind.

Although I can't think of a single instance when I gave away or threw away something that I later wished I had hung on to, it's still hard for me sometimes to give up an item I have treasured in the past. I always think maybe I'll lose enough weight to get back into that favorite skirt again, for instance. At one point in my life when I actually did succeed in dropping ten pounds, I gleefully dug out a pair of pants from a bottom drawer where I had been saving them, and drew the immediate and loudly voiced scorn of the peanut gallery I call a family because those pants were way out of style by then. Now I try to give away things before they're out of fashion, and I picture the people who will appreciate them and use them and love them. That far outweighs my selfish reluctance to release them from my closet.

Emotional junk is harder to unload. My skin is thinner

than I like to admit, and when someone hurts my feelings, I have a nasty tendency to cycle that around in my mind for a while, wondering what made them say what they did, what I could have done differently, what I should do now. I'm always a lot happier when I get it resolved, usually by talking with the person to clear the air, and then just let go of it.

In the Young Adult group that I was involved in during my college years, there was one particular girl whom I thought I knew quite well, but who seemed sort of distant and cold to me for several months in the middle of our acquaintance. One evening at a volleyball game, she came up to me and said, "I just wanted to tell you, I've been mad at you for about a year." Whoa. That one knocked me back a couple of steps. I wasn't sure how to respond, so I just said, "Really?" "Yeah," she said, and went on to tell me that she had heard I had said something hurtful about her to a third party and it had really upset her.

The incident was too far in the past for me to remember what I had or hadn't said, but by this time the third party in question had diminished in credibility enough that she had begun to question whether he had told her the truth or not. I felt terrible for this friend, who had carried this hurt around in her heart for so many months. Imagine feeling that wound afresh every time you ran into the person who had unintentionally inflicted it. Imagine the bitterness that would color all your associations with the group to which you both belonged. Imagine the amount of emotional energy wasted and stress built up around worrying whether that person would show up for an activity, what he or she would say, what "evidences" you could find that would justify your angry feelings toward the person. This is what happens when we don't get around to emptying our emotional Recycle Bin.

Here's another image that helps me understand this principle a little better. My husband and I try to pay off our credit card bill every month because I have this thing against paying interest. I hate it! It bugs me no end to pay extra money for something I've already used up. The absolute worst, though, is when I forget to pay the bill on time. Do you know that if you are even *one day* late with your payment, you have to pay not only the interest but a whole raft of other late payment penalties as well? This drives me crazy! So it's important to my well-being to pay attention and get that bill paid off promptly, so I don't have to think about it anymore.

I've discovered that there are a lot of times in my life when I pay "emotional interest." I have a nasty tendency to put off unpleasant tasks, especially when they involve a confrontation of some sort, and so I end up fretting about things that ought to have been taken care of long since. I carry the stress of the task around until it ends up costing me a lot more emotionally than it would have if I had just dug in and done it.

For example, one summer we were doing quite a bit of needed remodeling to our house in anticipation of a big family party we were going to host in August. A major part of the job was repainting, and we got the living room and the hall with all their trim done, but my husband wanted to use a higher-gloss paint on the doors opening into the hall, so we were saving those for last.

And save them we did! Somehow that task kept failing to surface on our to-do list, except sometimes when we were drifting off to sleep at night and one of us would mutter, "We've got to get those doors painted, honey," and the other one would grunt in agreement.

The closer we got to August, the sicker I felt about this job that simply had to be done. Finally, the week before the party, I told my husband to paint those doors or get a new wife. There were five of them: two bedrooms, a bathroom, and two closets, and his plan was to take them all off their hinges and line them up in the carport, roll the paint onto them, and let them dry outside overnight. That way he wouldn't have to be careful about the carpet, he could work more quickly, and the paint fumes wouldn't overpower the house quite so much.

Seemed like a great idea. The only problem was that by this point we were having to spend all our daylight hours putting the finishing touches on the yard, so he couldn't get started on the painting until after dark. This was no big deal to him: he owned a little spotlight contraption, and he figured I could play that light onto the doors while he applied the paint. Around ten o'clock that night he began removing the doors from the hinges and carrying them out to the carport.

We got everything set up, and I plugged in the light. Picture a late August evening in Utah. Can you guess what happened next?

Every mosquito, gnat, and other nocturnal insect within a five-mile radius seemed to get the word that something big was happening at the Watts house. The bugs came in droves, and the light gleaming off the surface of the first door as my husband rolled the paint onto it was an irresistible attraction for them. That door became, in effect, a giant slab of flypaper. After a few minutes of painting, picking off the bugs, and smoothing out the paint again, we saw that this was not going to work. My husband finally painted the doors by moonlight while I swished my arms around to try to keep the night life off them. It was not the happiest time in our married life.

Anyone can see how much less that job would have cost us if we had just gotten in and done it early on! Procrastination carries a heavy emotional price tag, but it's a hard habit to break. These days, if I find myself putting off a certain task repeatedly, I say to myself, "Is it time to paint the doors?" That usually snaps me out of it!

Another way we pay emotional interest is to continue harping on something long after the damage has been done and paid for. For the first several years of our marriage I had a bad habit of "keeping score," hanging on to grievances that I thought I could use as ammunition when we had an argument: "Well, I may have done *this,* but it's not as bad as when you did *that!*" The thing is, we had already fought about *that* and supposedly resolved it. By raising it again I was bringing into our present life the full weight of every argument we had ever had in the past. And in the meantime, I had been packing that emotional weight around with me. What a tragic waste of energy! What a lot of penalties to pay for errors long past that could have been gone if I hadn't insisted on clinging to them.

So, how can we avoid paying emotional interest? Since mistakes seem unavoidable, maybe we can minimize the damage by viewing them as learning experiences and then letting them go. This accomplishes two purposes: It takes the sting out of the mistake a little by investing it with some value, and it keeps us from making the mistake again.

One morning my son and I were walking out the door for school when we saw a skunk wandering up the middle of the street where we live. This was the closest I had ever been to a live skunk, and it was pretty interesting—until the creature took a sharp right turn and headed straight for our backyard! This might not have been so bad, except that our dog was out there. He started barking like a maniac on his side of the fence, which you would think would have scared the skunk off, but it was completely ineffectual. I would guess there must have been some little skunk babies in a nest under our shed in the backyard, because that skunk was not backing off. It coolly faced down the dog through the fence and took a fighting stance. I told my son to run in the front door and warn his father not to come out the back. I could just see him walking right into the middle of this battle!

Regrettably, we had to leave for school in order to make it on time, so we didn't get to see what happened, but we got the full story when we came home. My husband was in the shower when he got the skunk warning, so he jumped right out, threw on some clothes, and ran out to try to rescue the dog. He still had the towel with him, which he flapped at the skunk to frighten it off, but if a crazed, yapping dog didn't deter the animal, I don't know why he thought a damp guy waving a towel would do the trick. He did manage to get close enough to the gate to get hold of the dog, whereupon the skunk rushed into the backyard and dived under the shed; the dog yelped and ran into the house, rubbing himself on every piece of furniture and every square inch of carpet in an attempt to get rid of the stink; and my husband discovered that you don't actually have to be sprayed directly by a skunk to have its odor permeate your clothing, skin, and hair.

Scented candles aren't really much use in a situation like this one, but there were ten or fifteen of them lighted throughout the house when I got home from work that evening. We looked like a shrine of some sort. The next day, the nice people down at Animal Control gave us some chemical solution that worked pretty well to clean up the odor in the dog's coat and the man's skin. They also loaned us a trap, and we caught that skunk and another one a few days later—as well as our cat, who crawled into the box one evening to get shelter from a light snowstorm and ended up all crusted with eggshells and peanut butter.

A couple of weeks after all this brouhaha, my husband was out walking the dog when he (the dog, not my husband) lit out after something in the bushes a few dozen yards away. Sure enough, he came out yelping and stinking, so he earned himself another chemical bath. The difference between him and us was that we had learned by this time and didn't let him in the house until he was clean. The poor dog never did seem to catch on, and he got skunked again later on in the season.

Most of us, being smarter than that dog, can recognize a skunk once we've been sprayed by one. If we're wise, we'll stay away, no matter how tempting the offer. If we do happen to get sprayed, though, we'll clean up the mess as quickly as possible instead of keeping the smelly clothes around as a reminder of our stupidity. We may have missed on the "Just say no" front, but we can at least minimize the effects of the error if we can score some points in the "Just let go" category.

If you're having trouble unloading some things from your Recycle Bin, you might try asking yourself a couple of questions. If you are the one who has made a mistake, you can ask, "Have I done all I can to remedy the problem?" I remember one time when I had a misunderstanding with a friend, and I wrote her a letter explaining my thinking and apologizing for what I had done to hurt her feelings. It was hard to do, but I felt better afterward—a little better. An astute friend noticed me worrying over this a few weeks later and said, "You haven't really gotten that resolved, have you?"

"Sure I have," I said. "At least, I've done all I could. The ball's in her court now."

"No," said my friend. "You need to go see her."

"I sent her a letter."

"You need to go see her."

"I've said what I wanted to say," I insisted.

"Maybe you don't understand me," said my friend patiently. "You need to go see her and say it face to face. You need to look into her eyes and know that it's all right."

It was true. And it was hard, a lot harder than writing a letter, but I called and asked if I could come over, and I sat in this woman's living room and discussed with her what had happened. We cried together, we hugged, and we were truly friends again. Most important, I *knew* we were friends again. I didn't have to sit around wondering if I had been forgiven. However, only when I had truly done everything I knew how to do to fix the problem could I eliminate it from my Recycle Bin.

If someone else has committed the foul, and you're the one suffering from it, you might ask a different question: "Is this something that's likely to matter a year from now?" Chances are, no lasting damage has really been done, and you can save yourself a lot of time and stress by forgiving the person right away. Even professional basketball players get to foul six times before they're thrown out of the game—and the slate is wiped clean each time they play.

Most grievances fall in this "non-lasting" category. A few do not. Sometimes people need to make wholesale changes in their lifestyle in order to leave serious problems behind them. But the principle still holds true: what's past is past. Resist the urge to recycle all the old garbage; it really can be deleted from your life forever. The beauty of forgiveness is that it takes you forward from this point into a future that's bright and clean. This is true whichever end of the problem you are on.

If you're feeling particularly stressed, stop and take a good look at what you might be carrying around in your Recycle Bin. You'll be surprised at how much lighter you can feel if you just let go!

CHAPTER SIX

Look for the Answers in the Back of the Book

I recently came across an old calculus test booklet that I remembered having tucked away in college. I had gotten 100 percent on that test, but even then I sensed that, years hence, calculus would seem like a foreign language to me, and I wanted to hang on to some evidence that I had understood it once upon a time.

Now that my children are coming up into the algebra phase of their educational experience, I find with a little sadness that most of math is but a dim recollection for me. Rusty as I am, I'm not terribly confident when I try to lend a hand with their homework. One thing that helps a lot is that the textbook company often prints the answers to the odd-numbered problems in the back of the book. If I know where we're heading, it's easier for me to remember the steps that will get us there.

I used to wish that life came with answers in the back of

the book, at least to some of the questions. It seemed as if I could let go of a lot of stress if I could just relax about some things. I thought it would be really nice to be able to check my understanding on certain issues as I blundered ahead. Was I going in the right direction? Was I taking the right steps, in the proper order? These were questions that plagued me particularly in my young adult years, when it felt like most of the decisions I was making would affect the entire rest of my life and maybe even eternity. What if I messed up? Many was the time I wished for a few moments with a reliable crystal ball, just enough to reassure myself that things were going to turn out all right.

I'm grateful now that I didn't get that peek at my future. There seems to be some divine wisdom in the fact that life unfolds itself to us a little at a time. It's a system that allows us to enjoy events—or to endure them—as they happen, without becoming overwhelmed. We think we'd like to know where we're going, but I have to admit that if I had seen at age twenty the various turns my life would take in the next twenty years, I'm not sure I could have handled it. I sort of had to grow into those experiences—as do we all.

However, I have come to realize that, although we rarely get specific instructions, life is full of answers that keep us moving in the right general direction. If we can learn to recognize them, a lot of the burden we feel is alleviated. The trick is, they crop up in the most unlikely places. We really have to be listening.

For example, one evening my husband and I took our young children to a Chinese restaurant for dinner. Their experience with dining out had rarely extended beyond McDonald's, and they weren't happy with the atmosphere, the wait, or the cuisine. Suffice it to say, I did rather a lot of low-decibel scolding—hissing, to be more precise—during the course of that meal.

By the time the check came, I was frazzled, but not too weary to attack the fortune cookie that arrived with it on the little tray. My fortune, which could not have been more appropriate if my own mother had written it and placed it in my hands, said this: "An ounce of patience is worth a bushel of brains." That lesson, at that moment, was so profoundly right, it seared itself into my heart. I carried that little scrap of paper around in my wallet for several years to remind myself of a principle I really needed to understand.

Since then, I've always been faintly superstitious about fortune cookies, and I have saved many similar scraps of paper over the years. Usually they're just clever things I want to remember or hope for, like "A fascinating project is in your future," or "You will enjoy a well-deserved vacation." Sometimes they act almost like positive affirmations: "You generate enthusiasm in all around you." But once in a while, the miniature lesson wrapped up in that cookie is just what I need.

I'm thinking of another time, when I was suffering from having worn exactly the wrong thing to a luncheon social. The minute we walked in the door, I could see what I *should* have worn, but of course by then it was too late. I felt an almost uncontrollable urge to grab people and say, "I really do own a black sweater with gold spangles and a dramatically draping black skirt to go with it." Though I managed to resist that urge, I didn't feel any less a hick in my crisp white blouse and blue-patterned broomstick skirt, especially after someone brushed past me with a plate of ravioli and slimed up the sleeve of the blouse. I stood around feeling stupid for a couple of hours, consoling myself with bite-sized delicacies from the dessert buffet, and finally went home in a stupor of chocolate and low self-esteem.

The very next week I had Chinese food for lunch, and do you know what my fortune said? "Be yourself, and you will always be in fashion." It was not only an immediate consolation but also an inspiration to examine more closely who I really was and what I had to offer in any given situation, regardless of my wardrobe.

Herein lies the secret of fortune-cookie wisdom. The good folks of the Chang Noodle Company are not staying awake nights trying to come up with aphorisms that are going to change your life. However, you carry a lot of answers to your most serious questions right inside your heart, and if a fortune cookie can invite you to stop for a moment and take a look into that cache, you just might discover answers that were there all along.

It's not just fortune cookies that can work this way. A billboard, a song on the radio, the chance comment of a child—all kinds of everyday occurrences can unleash a thought process that will lead you to truths about yourself, if you're alert. I've heard these flashes of insight called "aha moments," and they can happen anytime.

I had one such moment years ago when I was driving to California with some friends. We stopped in Las Vegas for dinner, and my friend and I headed for the rest room together. We were in one of the fancier casinos, and the ladies' room was quite elegant, but what fascinated me most was a little vending machine that was dispensing, of all things, women's pantyhose. I had never seen such a thing, and I've never seen hosiery in a machine since then, but there they were, and we had to step closer to get a better look. After reading the label, my four-foot-ten friend looked up at me—I remind you that I am six feet tall—and burst out laughing. I saw right away what had struck her; the label proclaimed: "One Size Fits All."

"It's a lie!" my friend chuckled, and I had to agree, having worn many a pair of pantyhose in my day that ended up with the waistband slipping down and sort of binding my knees together, thus forcing me to shuffle home from church. Then it hit me that this was a lie that applied not just to pantyhose but to a broad range of life experiences. Much of the unhappiness I had felt as a student and later as a young mother had come from trying to fit into what I perceived as the perfect mold. I thought there was "one size" for the ideal life, and because it didn't always fit me, I sometimes felt lonely and out of synch.

The truth is, the gospel net gathers "of every kind" (Matthew 13:47), and you don't get thrown back into the sea for not having the right number of children or the right color of skin or the right amount of square footage in your house. One size does *not* fit all, unless we're talking about being clothed "with the bond of charity" (D&C 88:125) or having our "loins girt about with truth" (Ephesians 6:14).

That's a lot to learn from one simple label on a pair of pantyhose! Again, that lesson obviously was not on the manufacturer's packaging but in my heart, waiting to be thought about and recognized. If such answers can be unlocked by a chance reading of a label, what inspiration might be waiting within the pages of sacred scripture?

I have to confess that I have never had much luck with the time-honored practice of randomly opening my scriptures and finding the answer I was looking for right there on the page I happened to flip to. I usually end up in the maps section, which has frankly never held a whole lot of personal insights for my life, although I'm happy to know what countries the Apostle Paul traveled to on his Third Missionary Journey. The scriptures started yielding answers to me when I got serious about reading them for real on a regular basis.

The best advice I ever got in a Sunday School class was to keep a scripture journal. I tried this for a while and had a great experience. In a small notebook, I wrote down questions that occurred to me as I was reading. I wrote feelings about verses that struck a particular chord with me. The only problem was, I sometimes had trouble laying my hands on the notebook at the exact moment I was wanting to read, and I even started using that as an excuse to put off the reading. It's a sad but true commentary on the state of my life.

So, more recently, I picked up an inexpensive paperback copy of the Book of Mormon and tried writing those questions and feelings right in the margins, circling and underlining and starring things with a red pen. I could do this unhampered because I wasn't worried about "making a mess" in my fancier, leatherbound set. That system is working for me now, and if it stops working, I'll find something else, because when I'm consistent in my searching, I get answers from the scriptures that I never got before. There's not always an "aha" moment in every study session, but there is a gradual feeling of increased understanding of God's plan and my own place in it.

Here's an example to show what I mean. To place it in context, you should know that I have always, even as a child, been nervous about money. My mother clearly sensed this tendency in me, because I remember the day she sat me down and said, "Look, honey, if we ever sell the TV, you'll know we're in trouble. Until then, don't worry about it, okay?" The color television being the height of luxury in that era, I knew we must be safe if we could afford to own one. The fact that I needed that kind of reassurance as a ten-year-old child may give you some idea of the obsessive view I have had toward finances just about all my life.

Those feelings have sometimes made it tough to cope as an adult, especially since financial abundance never seemed to be part of the plan for us. In truth, we have always had plenty to meet our needs, but I couldn't always see that. Particularly in the early years of our marriage, I did a lot of fretting.

I used to work for several companies on a freelance basis out of my home, and I fell prey to the notion that if I just worked harder, put in a few more hours each week, we would get ahead financially. So I didn't say no to any job that came up. As deadlines started to crowd in on each other, I got more and more irritable and shoved my children further and further into the background. I knew it was pretty serious when I heard my two-year-old scolding her baby doll: "Not right now! Can't you see that Mommy is *working?*"

One day, in the middle of this mess, I came upon this scripture: "Wherefore, do not spend money for that which is of no worth, nor your labor for that which cannot satisfy" (2 Nephi 9:51). This brought me up short. I found myself asking, "Who am I doing this for, anyway?" It occurred to me that if I had been paying someone to watch my preschoolers, and they did it the way I was doing it at that time, I would have fired them and hired someone else. Walt Disney was a more important figure in those children's lives than their own mother!

That one scripture helped me sort out what was really of worth in my family's life, and I began to see ways in which I could labor that would be more satisfying. I didn't need to accept every project that was offered to me. I started to admit my time constraints up front, and if the clients still wanted me for the job, they would work within my schedule rather than the other way around. Some did, some didn't, but somehow, when the needs of my family came first in my heart, the work seemed to fall into place. Our family still had financial needs, and the children still had to make sacrifices sometimes when I had to get a project done, but the guilt on my part and the frustration on theirs was diminished because the purpose for the work was pure. The answer to that difficulty lay in the scriptures.

I recently got another answer for another set of circumstances. I was reading about Christ's visit to the Nephites in Third Nephi, chapter 11, which describes the people coming forward one by one to see and feel the prints of the nails and the wound from the spear in the Lord's side. That has always been a moving passage to me, as I contemplated his tremendous patience and the power of that experience for those witnesses. But this time through, these were the verses that leapt out at me: "And it came to pass that he spake unto Nephi (for Nephi was among the multitude) and he commanded him that he should come forth. And Nephi arose and went forth, and bowed himself before the Lord and did kiss his feet" (3 Nephi 11:18–19).

I loved Nephi in that moment. He had been the prophet whose preaching had likely saved many of those people from the destructions that swept their land when Christ was killed. He was their leader, their teacher, worker of miracles and raiser of his brother from the dead. What must he have felt when all his prophecies found their ultimate fulfillment in the coming of the Lord to his people? But he didn't push his way up to his "rightful place" at the front of the line. He didn't set himself up as the go-between or the man in charge of the group when Christ descended into their midst. He was just one of the believers, "among the multitude."

The Savior, however, knew him, and called him forth out of the crowd of thousands, and as I was thinking about what it must have been like for Nephi to hear his name spoken by the mouth of the Lord, a feeling came into my heart: "Emily, he knows your name, too." It wasn't a voice. It wasn't words spoken out loud so that I could hear them. It was just a quiet moment of understanding that God knows me as intimately as he knows Nephi and Joseph Smith and Moses and any of his other children whom he has called by name.

Do you know how many questions in my life are answered by that one bit of knowledge?

If this life is a test, I'd like to believe it is an "open-book" exam. Doesn't that just take a lot of the stress right out of it? What a relief it is to realize that we don't have to have all the answers memorized—we just have to know where to go to find them. It may take a lifetime and beyond to understand some things, but we can know now, today, that there is One who holds all the answers and will share them with us in his own way and time if we will keep looking for them.

CHAPTER SEVEN

Swallow Your Fears and Just Get in the Pool

My husband was sent on a work assignment to attend a convention in Las Vegas in early March one year, and he invited me to come along just to hang out in the sunshine and enjoy a little break from the routine. March in Utah being generally a gray and cold proposition, I was happy to accept the offer, and we drove, gloating, from soggy snowstorms into blue skies and eighty-degree temperatures. It was beyond gorgeous—it was healing, the promise of summer after a long, bleak stretch of winter.

On our first full day there, Larry headed off to the convention, and I lazed around the motel room for a while and then got into my swimsuit, thinking to get in a few laps in the beautiful pool I had glimpsed when we were checking in the night before. Because I don't put on my swimsuit within a fifty-mile radius of anyone who might recognize me, I don't have much occasion for wearing it, so I don't have a cute swimsuit cover-up to toss on over it for events such as this one. And I was too self-conscious to walk through the halls of the place in my ratty old bathrobe. So I threw on a T-shirt and a pair of jeans over the suit and wandered out to the pool. There it was, gleaming in the sunlight, even more inviting than it had been the previous night.

However, stationed around the pool, stretched out in lounge chairs and glistening with tanning lotion or cocoa butter—or canola oil, for all I knew—were several shapely, bronzed women, most of them accompanied by shapely, bronzed, equally slippery men. It having been a good eight years since any part of my body between my shoulders and my ankles had seen direct sunlight at all, I was somewhat intimidated by this.

I slipped quietly—inconspicuously, I hoped—over to an umbrella-covered table and set down my stuff: towel, can of pop, book to enjoy while lounging. I took a deep breath and pulled off the T-shirt, then stood there for several long moments, trying to summon the courage to step out of those jeans. I just couldn't bring myself to do it. I couldn't unveil those vast expanses of lily-white flesh in the stark brightness of the Las Vegas sun. I plopped into a chair and opened the book, pretending that had been my intention all along.

But it was a lie. I hadn't come to read. I could read at home, for heaven's sake—I had been reading at home all winter. I wanted to swim! The water was blue and calm and beautiful, but not a soul was in the pool. I would not be able to enter it unnoticed. I read the same paragraph of the book over and over again, the battle raging inside.

When a cartoon character is faced with a tough decision, he often gets a little good angel perched on one shoulder and a bad angel on the other, each advocating a certain course of action. In my case, it was more like an "angel of logic" that began whispering in my ear:

"You know, you're never going to see any of these people again."

True enough, I conceded.

"You know, they don't give a hoot what you look like; all they're concentrating on is what they look like."

That was probably true as well, I supposed.

"You know, even if they do take note of you, it will probably be just to recognize how great they look in comparison. What does it hurt you to give them that little ego boost?"

Thinking of it that way, and realizing how little thought was likely to be expended on a middle-aged, cellulite-ridden woman with phosphorescent thighs, I was able to shuck off those jeans and head for the pool. No way in the world was I going to jump in, though; I couldn't bear the thought of the splash. I stepped as nonchalantly as possible onto the first step—and realized in a flash why no one was in the pool. The proprietors of the motel hadn't bothered to heat the water. I suppose that when the customary 100-degrees-plus summer weather would hit Las Vegas a couple of months hence, there would be no need for an artificial pool heater, but I can tell you it was mighty cold on that early March day. I swam a couple of laps, teeth chattering, before I hauled myself out of there. My skin was more blue than white by then, but it didn't matter. I had won!

The moral of this little story is simple: Don't let your fears of what other people might think keep you from doing what you came here to do. Sometimes you've just got to take a deep breath and get in the pool!

This is admittedly hard to do sometimes. No one likes to have her weaknesses exposed for the whole world to see. I take some solace in the fact that most of the time the whole world isn't even paying attention in the first place. However, it only takes a couple of detractors to start that wheel of insecurity rolling. We are not helpless in the face of such circumstances; the stress can be diminished even during those times when a little scrutiny seems inevitable.

One easy thing to do is to deflect potential criticism by admitting your inadequacy right up front. If no one really expects you to do a thing right, they can't really fault you for doing it wrong. People are much more apt to be helpful than scornful if you give them a chance.

For example, once we were having an Enrichment Night class on how to crochet a little chick-shaped covering for a plastic Easter egg. I had always wanted to learn how to crochet, but having pretty much "flunked out" of the skill in Primary, where my friends all worked up darling vests and hats while I labored my way across one edge of a tea towel (a narrow edge, too), I didn't have much confidence. I got all the usual reassurances that experts love to give: "It's an easy stitch." "I taught my six-year-old granddaughter how to do this." "You can finish three of these in an hour." These are the same kind of people who say things like, "I can get anyone up on water skis." I hate to tell you how many times I have shattered that illusion for well-meaning boaters. So, although I didn't really expect that any of those claims would really apply in my case, I did think that in two hours' time I might be able to at least get a good start on a sweet little Easter chick.

I showed up eagerly for class, crochet hook and yarn in hand, and those women tried to teach me. Oh, how they tried! I don't know what is wrong with my fingers or my brain or whatever portion of my anatomy it is that prevents me from mastering nice handwork, but I kept hearing dark murmurs about "tension." Apparently, I am too tense to get the tension right when I crochet. Hence, whereas the pattern was intended to move in circles down the body of the upright egg, mine was coming out more like loose ovals that fit the egg only if we laid it on its side. I couldn't really see creating a "prone" chicken, so we decided instead to pronounce it a mouse, and my teachers even helped me attach two little round ears and a chain-stitched tail. We got a good laugh that evening and many times over the years as we remembered my custom-designed, handmade, chick-turned-rodent.

Sure, I felt a bit silly that I lacked the skill of a six-year-old with a crochet hook. But because I was good-natured and willing to try, and because I was willing to acknowledge my total dependence on someone else's skills, we accomplished something together that evening that would not have happened if I had fearfully stayed home. We may not have managed a suitable Easter decoration, but we created a bond.

Another thing you can do to take some of the stress out of a fearful situation is to prepare as much as you can beforehand. If you have to give a talk or perform a musical number, for instance, try practicing in front of a mirror. Read your talk out loud until you can hardly stand the sound of your own voice. Close your eyes and picture yourself in front of your audience, delivering your talk or music just the way you would hope to be able to.

If you're facing a teaching or interview situation that will involve interacting with others, it's helpful to make a list of as many questions as you can think of that people might ask. How would you answer them? Do whatever research you can to shore up your position. Know where you stand, and what your objective is, and you're less likely to be thrown off by people who don't agree with you.

I don't think our anxiety about performing in public ever really leaves us, no matter how much practice we have. I know that I have a recurring dream that visits me the night before any important situation I'm facing, even a big meeting at work or a concert one of my children will be participating in. I dream that I am on my way to the event, but something happens to prevent my getting there: the car breaks down, my ride doesn't show up, I run out of gas. The cause varies somewhat, but the effect is always the same—I find myself on foot, rushing frantically to the building, which I can see in the distance. As I'm working my way there, the streets become progressively seedier, and scary people start popping up around me. I begin darting from doorway to doorway, hiding from the bad guys and clutching my coat around me so no one can see my evening gown, which has somehow sprouted sequins by then to make me seem even more conspicuous and a greater target for muggers. I never get closer to the place where I'm supposed to be, but at least (so far) I've never been attacked. It's always a huge relief to wake up. Plus, I get the sense that whatever happens at the actual event, it can't be worse than not being able to get there at all!

That dream seems to be my subconscious mind's way of dealing with the "what-ifs." If you find yourself consumed with fears of what might happen, you can get your conscious mind into the act as well. The trick is to force those "what-ifs" into the category of the absurd. "What if I fell flat on my face on the way up the steps?" "What if I opened my mouth to start singing and a fly buzzed into it?" "What if the dry-erase marker exploded and spewed blue ink all over my white blouse?" "What if a big German shepherd sneaked into the building through a window and starting running up and down the aisles while I was talking?" "What if something triggered the automatic fire sprinklers and everyone in the room got sprayed down?" The little things that are actually more likely to go wrong seem so trivial in comparison to such scenarios that they lose some of their capacity to frighten us.

When it comes right down to it, worrying about a thing usually takes up more emotional energy than just getting in and doing it. Sometimes the best strategy is to take that deep breath and leap into the pool. I'm remembering an experience I had when I was at girls camp. I was twelve years old and a major klutz and, hence, afraid of pretty much anything physical. The prospect of the all-day hike made me nervous, but the event that was really turning me into an emotional wreck was the rock rappelling. There was a giant granite rock on the premises, and each cabin of girls was to have a turn to rappel down the face of it. Our turn wasn't until Friday, the last full day of camp, so I had an entire week in which to ponder this pending activity, which I did with the greatest dread. I thought of playing sick, but I didn't want to miss arts and crafts and the other things that were planned for the day.

I had a great time all week, but always Friday loomed in the back of my mind, waiting with its imminent peril. When it finally came, I was almost sick for real. But I followed my cabin-mates out to the top of the rock, graciously ushering them all ahead of me in the line (a trick I had learned in sixth grade when we were doing tumbling and I couldn't seem to master a simple forward roll). My hands were shaking so badly by the time I got up to the front, I could barely tie the knot in the rope that was going to support me. Our counselor, Tibs, spoke gently to me, reminded me of what to do, helped me get everything secured, and sent me over the top of the cliff to my sure death (or so I thought). One step, two, and three, and I suddenly realized that this was great! This was a lot of fun! I wasn't going to get smashed into the side of the rock. I wasn't going to fall. I could do it!

I can still remember with a flush of triumph the way I felt as I climbed back over the top of that rock.

When we take on something that's hard for us, and we conquer it, it builds a kind of strength inside that will see us through other tough times. My dad taught me a little lesson in this one day when we were having lunch at a cafeteria and he selected a bowl of cottage cheese. I had heard him speak disparagingly about this particular food on more than one occasion, so I expressed some surprise. "I thought you didn't like cottage cheese, Dad," I said.

"I don't," he answered.

"Well?"

"Oh," he said, "sometimes I eat something I really don't like, just to show myself that I can do it. It builds character."

If that's true, our daughter who is serving a mission in Africa is brimming with character. I have the photos to prove that she sampled a plate of caterpillars one day—a delicacy that she describes as definitely *not* "slimy yet satisfying." More important, she and her missionary brother have done many other difficult things that have helped prove to them how much they are capable of accomplishing. They wouldn't have chosen for themselves many of the circumstances they face, but they have learned to push past their fears and just do what they came to do.

This illustrates one of the greatest deterrents to fear,

which is to be firm in your purpose. If you know what you want to accomplish, and move forward with the determination that you are *going* to accomplish it, the obstacles that inevitably arise will not keep you from your goal.

I have experienced many times in my life when it seems impossible for me to achieve what I need to. The task is too great, the time is too short, the stumbling blocks are too plentiful, and I can't get my mind around how the thing is going to get done. I have come to call such times "Gideon moments." I love the story of Gideon in the Old Testament (Judges 6–8), in which the Lord, wanting to prevent the Israelites from taking credit for their own victory in their battle with the Midianites, winnows down their army from 32,000 to 300. In the mathematics of the world, 300 men are never going to prevail against a host that is "like grasshoppers for multitude" (Judges 7:12). It just doesn't compute. But when the Lord fights on your side, you win. It's that simple.

Will he fight on your side? If your determination is to serve him with all your heart, might, mind, and strength, he will—every time. We are supported in all that we do by forces we never see. We are like the servant of Elisha, who cried, "Alas, my master! how shall we do?

"And he answered, Fear not: for they that be with us are more than they that be with them.

"And Elisha prayed, and said, Lord, I pray thee, open his eyes, that he may see. And the Lord opened the eyes of the young man; and he saw: and, behold, the mountain was full of horses and chariots of fire" (2 Kings 6:15–17).

May our eyes be opened, that we might see and understand how much depends on our going forth and doing what we came to do. When we are true to our purpose and trust the Lord to make us better than we could ever be on our own, our fears will melt away. Like Gideon, we will march forward with our little army of resources and conquer!

CHAPTER EIGHT

Stretch,
Don't Snap

For about a year when he was too young to get a better job, one of our sons undertook to cover a newspaper route. As usually happens, this became a family affair, especially on the weekends when there were several sections to collate and the papers were too heavy for him to carry on his bike. We spent many bleary-eyed Sunday mornings stacking, folding, and trying to get the little rubber bands to stretch all the way around the expanded weekend editions of the paper. Often the elastics would break as we were putting them on, which was bad enough, but occasionally they would wait to snap until the kid tossed the paper up onto the porch. This was much worse, since the newspaper would virtually explode, scattering sections across the steps and sometimes under the porch railing into the yard. We would have to stop, gather everything back up, and try to make the paper presentable. We could have been a lot more efficient if those cheapo rubber bands had just had a little more stretch to them.

Similarly, I have encountered many situations in life where a little more flexibility would have served me well. I have learned that I can save myself a lot of stress by stretching instead of snapping.

This has not come naturally to me. I have a long history of fussing over stuff. For example, when our local amusement park was making the switchover from individual ride tickets to an all-day pass, I spent the first couple of summers adding up ticket prices in my mind to make sure my kids were getting the full value out of their passes. This ridiculous behavior reached its peak when we were on our way out of the park one year and I insisted on dragging the kids on "one more ride" that was right there close to the exit. They were tired and beyond ready to go home, but this was an eight-ticket ride that would really cement the value of that admission pass and prove to me that we hadn't wasted money.

The only problem was, it was a spook alley ride that was geared to teens instead of young children—you know the kind, with wax-museum-type figures cutting off people's heads and climbing out of coffins and the like. My poor little preschoolers were completely traumatized by those visual images. The whole way home, all they could talk about was "that scary ride Mom made us go on." All the fun of that long day had dissipated because I had to get in another couple of bucks' worth of ride. This experience demonstrates that mine is not a particularly flexible personality.

That's odd, too, because I certainly wasn't raised to be uptight about such things. Both of my parents are extremely calm, reasonable people. In fact, one of the stories of greatest amusement in our family folklore is the account of a day when our mother had just plain had enough, and she stomped through the living room muttering, "Five pigs and one slave! That's all we have in this house!" My father, upon hearing this tale of woe, said with a hurt look on his face, "*Five* pigs?" (There are only four children in my family.)

Dad himself has a matching story, an incident that occurred on a family vacation. My father is a tall man, six-foot-seven, and motel beds don't provide a great rest for him, so I suspect he was a little close to the edge to begin with. We were in a small convenience store choosing items for a quick breakfast when my younger brother acted up one too many times, and my dad swatted him on the bottom. My brother was so astonished he lost hold of the piece of fruit he had selected, and he cried out indignantly, "You made me drop my peach!" This got the attention of everybody in the store! We fell apart laughing, partly because we were so glad to see our brother get what he deserved, but mostly because it was so completely uncharacteristic for my father to lose his temper that way. The fact is, if you have a history of stretching, it seems pretty funny when you do occasionally snap.

Anyway, those being the only instances of snapping on my parents' part that I can really remember from my growing-up years, I clearly have no one to blame but myself for my own tendency to be rigid. I have come only gradually to the understanding that my life is a lot less stressful when I am able to bend a little.

Of course, there are some areas in which there is no compromise and never will be. If the cashier accidentally rings up green grapes when I have bought the more expensive red ones, I will hold up the line and make her charge me more, because I know I simply can't enjoy eating those grapes if I got them under false pretenses. There are moral laws that our family cannot violate in the least degree if we want to be happy, and we will hold firm on those.

However, there doesn't seem to be any rule on the eternal books that says we have to be on time for every social event we attend, so I have learned that it's all right to be flexible when my husband pulls his inevitable stunt of running upstairs and jumping into the shower five minutes before we're supposed to be pulling out of the driveway. I prefer to be prompt. But if it comes down to a choice between arriving ten minutes late and cheerful or on time and furious, I'll go for the former. This is not worth fighting about.

Being late isn't really what makes me snap. Frankly, usually no one cares—and if I know it's going to be a big deal, I just give my husband a target departure time fifteen minutes before the actual deadline so that I don't have to pace up and down in the hall outside the bathroom calling through the door, "Are you hurrying?" We generally aren't brought to the snapping point by what actually happens but by what we *expected* to have happen. So I find that I snap less if I just set my expectation meter a little lower. It's like resetting your water-heater thermostat when you have small children so they won't accidentally scald themselves. If you lower your expectations when it's appropriate to do so, you're less likely to get burned.

For example, if I came home with a bill from the car repair shop for eighty dollars for an oil change and lube job, my husband would go through the ceiling, because his expectation would be more in the neighborhood of thirty to forty dollars. But when something under his car's hood exploded in my parents' driveway and leaked all over the place, and we had to have the car towed down to that self-same repair shop, and the bill for fixing it was eighty dollars, we were relieved beyond measure. Only eighty dollars! What a blessing! The issue, you see, is not one of paying eighty dollars to the car repair shop. It is totally a matter of expectations.

When I was a child, my parents took me to the Salt Lake Tabernacle to hear a performance of Handel's *Messiah*. The words were printed in the program, and when I read them through as we waited for the concert to get under way, I was encouraged by their brevity. "Hallelujah! For the Lord God omnipotent reigneth. The kingdom of this world is become the kingdom of our Lord and of his Christ, and he shall reign for ever and ever, King of kings, and Lord of lords." It takes all of thirteen seconds to read. How was I to know that it represented more than five minutes of music? Reading along, I thought I would scream when they kept singing the same thing over and over again! It was another classic case of expectations being at odds with reality, and I'm afraid I didn't get much out of that cultural experience because I was just too mad.

Life is unpredictable enough that we can't always get what we expect. It's helpful to have some resources in reserve for when the unexpected does rear its ugly head. Because our family owns three motor vehicles, for instance, with no fewer than 50,000 miles on any of their odometers, we know that we're going to have some auto maintenance bills each year. We don't know how many. We can't predict what's going to go wrong next. Until I learned to set aside a small reserve fund for such emergencies, I used to fall apart every time one of the cars did. Now, although I hate paying money just to get a car running normally again, I can be a lot more philosophical about it—because it no longer throws my budget off for the next two months if I suddenly have to replace my brakes.

On a much lesser scale, I have learned to hide away extras of items that have a bad habit of disappearing in our house: scissors, rolls of tape, hairbrushes, pens with actual ink in them, calculators, nail clippers. I keep a little emergency box of such things so that I don't have to scream at the children when I can't lay my hands on something that I need in a hurry. (And doesn't it seem like you always need tape in a hurry?)

Sometimes you head into a day or week knowing up front that it is going to be tough. The pioneers had a strategy for that: Circle the wagons. There are times in a family's life when it pays to get everybody together and solicit the cooperation of each individual member—"circle the wagon" times.

We had a whole month like that recently, when somehow my husband and I both ended up getting scheduled to be out of town more than once in the same month, and a couple of times our absences overlapped. We gathered the children in a family council and told them exactly what was up and that we would really need their help to keep things together. We wrote down clearly on a large calendar the various dates we would be traveling and brainstormed what we could put in the freezer to have ready for quick meals and what the kids would do on the evenings we had to be gone. It was a hard month for everyone, but we got through it all right because we had marshaled our resources carefully right up front.

This strategy of reserve resources is also important if you ever have to go anywhere with small children. Chances are, you'll need as many resources as you can muster. Start with realistic expectations: Are you really going to be able to spend three hours at the mall with a three-year-old and a baby? What are the chances that they're both going to fall asleep peacefully in the double stroller? What will you do if the three-year-old refuses to sit in the stroller and instead insists on pushing it through the crowded aisles all by herself? What if the baby screams to be carried? We endured many a shopping trip in our early parenting days with a toddler on Daddy's shoulders, an infant in Mom's arms, and a stroller full of shopping bags. If you have to take children shopping, try to team up with another responsible adult. This is like putting two elastic bands on the Sunday paper— it distributes the pressure so that neither of them breaks.

Also, plan for restroom breaks and food stops, and try to go into at least one store that would hold some interest for your child.

Keeping options open is another way to increase your stretch quotient. Sometimes it's possible to give a fussy child a choice: "We can just go straight home right now, or we can shop for fifteen more minutes and then go get an ice-cream cone on the way home." Be careful with this one, though, and be sure you offer choices you can live with. If you're really not in a position to go home until you finish the shopping, modify the selection list: "Shall we go into three more stores, or only two?"

Little children aren't the only ones who behave better if they have choices. I've noticed with teenagers that they don't really care much for being told what to do. It's not that they're unwilling to do it, necessarily—they just seem to have a thing against being "ordered around."

So we try to give our teenage children a lot of leeway to set their own schedules and plan their own lives. They know what we feel is important: church and school attendance, homework, appropriate dating behavior, helping out in the family. We tell them they start out with an "A" in trust from us. Whether they keep that "A" or not is up to them. We don't impose many restrictions on them unless they demonstrate that they need them by letting that "trust grade" slip.

So far, they've all been willing to work hard to maintain our trust, knowing that it's to their benefit to do so.

With our teenagers, we try never to say no if yes is a possibility at all. That way, when we *do* have to put our foot down, they understand that it's not a capricious decision. They're not at the mercy of our bad mood or their own poor timing in making a request. We make it plain that we trust them to make good choices, to be honest with us about what they're doing, and to communicate with us often about their lives. Then we pretty much turn them loose to go forward and do. I can't say whether this strategy would work in every family, but it has served us well, and so far we have had a great time with all our teenagers.

Having a variety of options: it works for small children, for teenagers, and for adults, too. It can clear the way for you to get to do *something* even if you can't do everything. If Larry and I planned to go to dinner and a movie, for instance, and one of us got hung up at work and couldn't get away in time, we wouldn't scrap the whole evening. We might choose a later movie, or maybe we'd just grab a quick bite on the way to the theater and then go out afterward. If the goal is to have a good time, rather than to do specific things in a specific order, it's easier to be flexible, because there are lots of ways to accomplish that goal.

A willingness to be flexible can actually lead you to

unexpected fun. One weekend we decided on the absolute spur of the moment to take a little overnight trip to a city a couple of hours north of our home. There was a play running in their community theater that we wanted to see, and we were feeling an urge to get out of town, to shake loose from our regular routine. We came home from work Friday night, explained the plan to the kids, and were in the car and on our way Saturday morning. We spent the day at a gorgeous lake and returned to our motel in town just in time to catch a huge parade of classic cars driving up and down Main Street. That seemed like more fun to the majority of family members, so we traded the play for the parade and a swim in the motel pool. The next day we went to church with some friends who lived in that city, and then drove home. We had been away all of thirty-six hours, but it felt like a week's vacation! That little bit of stretching in our lives prevented a lot of snapping down the road.

Of course, you wouldn't want to run every family vacation on those terms. Some opportunities have to be planned well in advance. All I'm suggesting is that we not program our lives so completely that we can't tolerate any variance— because life is going to throw us a curve ball once in a while, and we have to be able to take it.

Believe it or not, though, planning can actually be a key ingredient in spontaneity. It's easier to be flexible if you're crystal clear in your own mind about what it is really important for you to accomplish in a given day. I do best when I choose the top three things that simply, positively *have* to be done, and make sure I find time for them. If the rest of the day falls to pieces, I can still feel some degree of peace when I crawl into bed, knowing that I accomplished the most vital tasks. And if I get more done than I expected, it feels like a real bonus!

If you feel like you're operating right on the brink of snapping, stop and take a look at what you might do to stretch a little in some areas. Shore up your resources if you can, remembering that it's all right to ask for help and that someone else could likely take over part of the load you're carrying. Decide if you're making an issue over things that aren't really worth fighting about. See if your expectations could be adjusted in a way that would make everyone happier. And above all: Relax! If you can't get away for an overnight break, how about at least a leisurely bubble bath with some soothing music playing in the background? Add a couple of chocolates on the side and watch the stress melt away!

CHAPTER NINE

Watch Out for Crossed Wires

When our son was three, he went through a phase when we could not get him to pray. He wouldn't participate when we had family prayers, and he wouldn't say his own individual prayers, either. I chalked it up to three-year-old stubbornness and opted not to turn it into a power struggle, but after this had gone on for a couple of months, I began to worry. One day I finally asked him outright why he wouldn't pray anymore.

"Oh," he said matter-of-factly, "I don't like Heavenly Father."

"Really?" I said, trying hard not to overreact. "Why not?"

"Well," he replied, "Heavenly Father came to our Primary in a box, and he was scary."

It was suddenly all clear to me. Our creative Primary presidency had rigged an appliance box with Christmas lights and dials to look like a time machine, and every now and then they would do a "Back to the Scriptures" role-play for Sharing Time. On the day in question, "Moroni" had been the featured guest, portrayed by a gentleman with a full head of snowy white hair, wearing a white robe.

My little Sunbeam never got past that costume. To him, white hair plus white robe equalled Heavenly Father, and the booming voice and immediate presence of supposed deity in the Primary room was beyond his capacity to bear. No wonder he didn't want to pray—what if that person showed up at our house!

This illustrates that different people interpret reality differently, based on their frame of reference. This crossing of wires happens all the time, and yet we tend to assume that because we're all speaking the same language, we're understanding things the same way. I'm here to tell you, it just ain't so.

Part of the problem with communicating in English is that many words have more than one meaning. This can be particularly confusing for children, who know what they're trying to say even if the adults in their lives can't quite understand them. Our son bounded into his grandmother's house one fall day, for example, and asked point-blank, "Grandma, do you have any hang-ups?" She sputtered around for a minute as my husband and I exchanged horrified looks, until our little boy went on, "'Cause I want to hang up my coat." Whew! Thank goodness we figured out what he was really asking before Grandma launched into a description of any psychological problems she may have been experiencing!

We had a similar problem with a homework assignment another son was trying his best to complete on his own one evening. He was supposed to define the "bold" words on the page, and it seemed to be taking him way longer than it ought to have. He finally came to me in tears, saying, "I've read and read, but I can't find any words that mean *strong* or *courageous!*" Poor kid! As soon as I explained the concept of bold-faced type, he had the thing done in a flash.

A lot of the stress in our lives seems to spring from such crossed wires. We think we're communicating perfectly clearly, but somewhere along the way the message has gotten garbled. My husband and I had a standing argument for several years over one such communication problem.

I don't remember how or with whom it started, but the argument arose over what was meant by the designation "next Friday." To Larry, "next Friday" meant "the next Friday we come to," whereas to me, it meant "the Friday of next week." So, for example, if it were Monday, October 7, "next Friday" to Larry would be the eleventh, but to me it would be the eighteenth. The eleventh would be "this Friday" in my book.

This gets harder and more confusing depending on the day of the week. If it's Thursday, for example, "next Monday" might mean the same thing to both of us (being both the next Monday we come to and the Monday of next week). But if it's Tuesday, "next Saturday" isn't quite clear, even though there are the same number of days between Tuesday and Saturday as there are between Thursday and Monday. Are you thoroughly confused yet? So were we, to the extent that we began polling family members and friends in search of support for our varying positions on the issue. We found a fairly even division of opinions.

There's an easy way to avoid the stress of this miscommunication altogether, of course, a way that we have long since adopted. We make a habit of saying, Friday, the eleventh, or Friday, the eighteenth, rather than *this* or *next,* and we double check our perceptions to be sure the other person has understood. This is not hard to do, once you know it needs to be done. My suggestion is to assume it needs to be done, not just with *this* and *next* but with other important communications as well. Clarify whenever possible, and ask questions to be sure the other person understands, and everyone will probably be a lot happier.

This is sometimes hard to do, especially in a marriage. We've been raised with the fantasy that two people who are really in love understand each other perfectly. It's no surprise that a staple element of romance novels and movies is the hero who knows exactly what the heroine wants, sometimes before she even knows it herself.

In one romantic comedy film I saw a few years ago, the heroine was determined to find the man she was fated to marry, who had a specific name she had been "told" by a Ouija board and later by a gypsy fortune teller. The poor shoe salesman who fell in love with her but had the wrong name became her supposed ally in her quest to find Mr. Right. The night she had a date with the man she thought was "the one" (although it was actually a set-up), this real true love of her life presented her with a pair of shoes to go with her outfit. Of course, they were perfect. They were the right size, the right color, and exactly the right style to complete her ensemble. Be honest, now—do you know any man in real life who could pull that off?

We suffered for years because I thought that Larry should be able to surprise me on my birthday. If he really loved me, I thought, he would know what I wanted for my birthday without my having to ask for it. I even got the crazy idea in my head that if I had to tell him, it didn't count. I had a lot of rather unhappy birthdays as a result, and Christmas was no picnic either.

The other side of that coin was that he *never* wanted to be surprised. If we were going to spend money for a present, he was going to make darn sure it was something he wanted. Most of the time he would go out and buy it for himself before the big day, because what was the sense in waiting when he already knew what he was going to get? This took a lot of the joy out of it for me. Half the fun of Christmas is seeing your loved one's eyes light up when he discovers that you got him the perfect gift! Or at least, that's what I always supposed.

Twenty-five years later, we have reached a reasonable accord. The rule is, I go with him to pick what I want for my main present, but he has to get me at least one present that I don't know about, with a maximum value of twenty-five dollars. Plus, he has to throw in dinner at a restaurant for my birthday. I get to spend twenty-five dollars on birthday or Christmas surprises for him, with the understanding that he will pick out the rest of what he wants, and I generally cook his favorite foods for his birthday meal.

I've given up measuring my husband's love for me in terms of his ability to read my mind. I've found out it's much easier to just ask for what I want. He's perfectly happy to take out the garbage, for example, but a lot of the time it simply doesn't occur to him. I've seen him balance a family-sized cereal box on top of a full load in the kitchen can and walk away satisfied because it didn't fall. Believe me, this isn't worth fighting about. Ask and ye shall receive—and if ye thank, ye may receive again the next time without even having to ask.

The difference between asking and nagging, I think, has something to do with the expectation behind the request. I find that if I merely ask my husband for help, without implying that it is his duty to pitch in or that it is a burden for me to have to ask, it goes over better. It also helps to frame a request specifically. I have asked for help to get the kitchen cleaned up in a hurry before the dinner guests arrive, only to find him scouring out the inside of the microwave. It works better to say, "Could you please come in here and do the floor while I'm finishing up the counter-tops?"

This works with children, too. Sometimes it takes a little exploration and fine-tuning to get the communication down, but it can be done. Case in point: We started the school year with a rule that the kids had to leave word where they could be reached if they weren't going to be home when I got home from work. Everyone was happy to do this, but we kept running into problems. Occasionally they forgot, and there had to be a consequence imposed to help them over-come that. More frequently, though, they would tell one of their other siblings where they were going, and that sibling would forget to tell me, or would be gone as well, so the word never filtered all the way down to me. We discussed this and clarified the rule: You have to write on the white board where you are, or, if you go straight to a friend's house from school, you have to leave a message on the answering machine. It's the same rule, with the same intent, but communicated in such a way that it is within anyone's power to obey.

This principle applies down the line. If you say, "Clean your room," it is always helpful to check the child's perception of what is meant by a "clean room." If you don't want to find piles of debris shoved under the bed, or a layer of dust thick enough to stuff a pillow with, be specific.

If you get a negative reply to the question, "Do you have any homework?" you may want to follow it up with, "Do you have any homework that you know about that's not due tomorrow?" This will save you a lot of stress two weeks down the road when the science term project suddenly appears on the child's radar screen the night before it is due.

Don't expect that children understand things on an adult level. They just don't have the frame of reference. You would never tell an adult the plot of a movie you were about to see, for instance, because it would spoil the suspense. But a child, particularly a small child, might actually enjoy the movie more if he or she knows what to expect. If you question the truth of this, keep track of how many times in a row your little one asks to watch the same video. We went through a *Cinderella* phase that almost did me in, but my little girl loved it. This demonstrates the value of crystal-clear communication. Children who know what to expect are less likely to be disappointed—or to disappoint you.

Our son threw a loop into his nursery leader's plans one day when she had prepared a lesson she thought would be interesting to the children. The topic was something along the lines of "Heavenly Father created animals," and she had caught an ant and put it in a container to bring to class. This, being November, wasn't as easy as it sounds. She released the ant onto the table, but before she had a chance to explain her purpose, my little helper cried, "Oh, an ant!" and pounded his fist right down on it. So much for respect for nature and the beauty of creation. I know the teacher wanted to surprise the children, but it might have been more effective to bring them all on board regarding the significance of the ant before releasing the unsuspecting creature into their midst.

Another aspect of communicating clearly with children is teaching them that not all communication is to be trusted equally. Come to think of it, we might need a little practice understanding this even as adults. My husband and I attended several vacation resort and time-share presentations before we caught on that the fabulous prizes being offered weren't as grand as they seemed. The 35mm camera, for example, broke apart in our hands before we had even left the premises. The "free" vacation required only a $150 reservation fee. The barbecue grill was barely large enough to accommodate two hamburgers. We hit on a winner or two in the course of things, but by and large we would have been better off to skip the presentations entirely.

Most of our children have gone through a phase where they have been enchanted by television infomercials. They are completely convinced that the product they have been watching for half an hour is the answer to all my home-making ills. I've gone so far as to buy a few things from the "As Seen on TV" store in our local mall, just to demonstrate to them that things are not always as they appear.

I thought I had taught my children to hang up on telephone solicitors with a polite, "We're not interested, thank you." So you can imagine my surprise at receiving a congratulatory note in the mail regarding the new phone service I had signed up for. This was news to me! I called the service number immediately, and when they checked their records they found that they had sold the service to my thirteen-year-old son. I'm sure that when they called, they asked if he was empowered to make decisions regarding the family's phone service, and I'm equally sure that he had no idea what they were asking and just answered yes to everything without thinking about it.

Advertisers seem particularly skilled at manipulating language to make it serve their purposes. They can tell the truth even while conveying something quite different. If you're in the habit of scanning your snack-food packaging for the calorie count, for instance, be sure you keep reading to the part that tells you how many "servings" are in the package. It's pretty annoying to be consuming what you thought were 160 calories' worth of baby doughnuts, only to find that the package contains 480 calories!

My favorite advertising claim, though, was one shared with me by my friend Christine. She confided that she had bought a new antiwrinkle cream that promised younger-looking skin. "When I tried it," she said, "it made my face break out all over." Then she added, thoughtfully, "I guess, technically, it told the truth. It gave me the skin of a teenager!"

Intentionally or not, wires get crossed. To eliminate the stress this causes, check your communication level carefully, be wary of false communications, and try to relax and laugh it off when things don't go exactly as planned. It probably won't be the end of the world if an ant ends up smashed on the table once in a while!

CHAPTER TEN

Play the Music Life Gives You

I have sung with the Utah Symphony Chorus off and on for more than a decade, and in that time the one piece we have repeated most often has been Beethoven's Ninth Symphony. Some people claim to be tired of it, but I never feel that way. Singing it is an amazing experience every time.

One of the things I look forward to in rehearsing the Ninth is to get to the final week, when they add the soloists to the mix. This is a piece that requires great solo work, and I love to see who's been invited. There have been all different styles of voices, but I have rarely been disappointed.

As important as the soloists are to the success of the performance, however, this is also a piece that can't be done without a choir. That great cry of joy takes at least a hundred people to pull it off properly. And when you're singing at the top of your lungs from the bottom of your heart, in a crowd of other singers who are doing the same thing, it is a magical feeling.

One evening the thought struck me, what if there weren't a choir part to this piece? What if people like me, who are reasonably competent but don't have the pipes to do those big solo numbers, never got to participate in the great music of the world? What a loss it would be in my life if there weren't a way for me to make a contribution on a "lesser level"!

Then another thought occurred to me. What if they couldn't find a hundred people willing to sing in nonsolo roles? What if people thought, "Well, I can't be the soloist, so I'm not going to sing at all." Think how much poorer the musical world would be!

I'm grateful to live in a time and place where all sorts of life experiences are available to suit all sorts of people. And one thing I love about the Church is that most people get a chance to have experiences all along the spectrum. One year you might be like the orchestra conductor, and preside over a whole organization, and the next you might be like one of the violins, a teacher or a committee member. Either way, you can grow and thrive—but not if you're mad that you got assigned to the violin section and insist on playing the oboe part instead!

I find that the times I am most out of harmony with myself are the times when I have been unwilling to play the music that's in front of me. Coincidentally, this happens to cause me some of my greatest stress in life as well. Let me give you a few examples to show you what I mean.

For years, it seemed as if we were always playing "catch-up ball" on our finances. Whenever we got a little windfall, like a tax return or a Christmas gift of cash, it got sucked right down into the black hole to pay for something or other. Nothing ever boosted us ahead.

Determined one night to get to the bottom of this, I sat down with a book on budgeting and went through the whole exercise it suggested of tracking three months' worth of checks to see where our money was going, and comparing that with the money we had coming in. You probably won't be surprised to learn—though it surprised me—that our outlay was just slightly larger than our income. We were not deeply in debt, but we were kind of drifting along accumulating a little obligation here and there, which deficit then acted like a sponge for any extra money that came in. When I took a good look at the truth, it was clear that we needed to either make more or spend less. But we hadn't been playing from the music on our stand; we had been spending what we *thought* we should be able to spend, based on what we made, without ever planning for contingencies. Things went a lot more smoothly for us when we lived according to our true circumstances, as hard as that adjustment was. It was up to us to change the music we'd been given, if we could, but in the meantime we needed to buck up and work with what we had.

Can you see how stressful it can be to refuse to live with reality? We can alleviate a lot of that stress by taking a good, hard look at life and figuring out how to operate in harmony with the way things are instead of moaning that they aren't the way they ought to be.

Here's another example: When my children were little, I used to dream about how much easier my life would be when they grew up a bit and went off to school. I longed for the unbroken blocks of time, the peace to do whatever projects I wanted to without little hangers-on wanting to "help," the freedom to eat a chocolate doughnut in the middle of the morning without having to buy half a dozen more to share.

Then, when the kids *did* go off to school, I missed the less-structured days when we could just pick up and go to the zoo or the mall and not have to worry about homework or parent-teacher conferences or who was being mean at recess this week. I missed being able to stay out later at night instead of rushing home to get the kids in bed so they wouldn't be too tired for school the next day. I missed the days when their biggest trial had been Mom making them take a bath.

See, there are great things about preschool days and great things about school days. But if you're constantly looking over on the other person's music stand, coveting the music that you'll probably get to play someday, you can completely miss your own part today—and you'll never get that part back. When I was single, I wanted to be married. After I got married, I longed for the freedom of my single days. And so on, and so on.

Now that I know this about myself, I'm trying to make a more conscious effort to enjoy life right where I am today. I can look at any five-year interval in my life and recognize the many changes that have taken place, so I'm pretty sure life will be different for me five years from now. I won't ever be this age again, or have children this age, or be working on these particular projects. I need to learn what I can from them, and enjoy all the wonderful things about them, before I move on.

Of course, it's not enough just to be satisfied with the music that's in front of us. We've got to get in there and *play* it. Many people sit quietly through the symphony of life, hoping no one will notice that they're not really playing their instruments, keeping still for fear that they might hit a sour note or come in on the wrong beat or something. If a musician in a professional orchestra did that, he or she would be fired! We didn't get sent to earth to sit passively in the audience while other people live their lives in front of us. If we don't play our part, the music will be diminished.

The story of the widow's mite teaches us that it's not how much we give, but the heart with which we give it that counts. My daughter had an experience on her mission that vividly illustrates this principle. Walking down the street in Zimbabwe, a small country in southern Africa, she and her companion often encountered street children begging for food or money. They tried to carry very little with them, as their mission president had instructed them not to begin a cycle of giving that would never end. So our daughter had devised a clever answer, and when she was approached by a young boy one day she pulled a face and said, "I'm sorry! I haven't eaten today either! Haven't *you* got anything for *me?*" He looked at her solemnly for a moment, and then reached into a tattered pocket, pulled out a few coins, and held them out to her. That got her right in the heart, and she reported, "I couldn't help it; I gave him everything I had."

Those children owned next to nothing, but they took care of each other. As long as one person was eating, they would all eat. Doesn't that sound a little like Zion to you?

We need never withhold our giving out of fear that we're not giving enough. I had a great experience at the Brigham Young University Women's Conference one year that showed me this. We had heard from a speaker who was a native of eastern Europe, and she had detailed for us some of the difficulties of a woman she knew there who was trying to save up enough money for a serious operation. After the speech, someone stepped up spontaneously to the microphone and suggested, "Sisters, if each of us gave one dollar, we could send this sister home with enough money for her friend's operation." Purses flew open all over the Marriott Center, and self-appointed volunteers started down the aisles gathering up the money. It was a tangible reminder to me that if everyone gives a little, it quickly adds up to a lot. If I remember correctly, they collected more than $15,000 that day—one dollar at a time. But that wouldn't work if people thought one dollar was too insignificant to be worth giving.

Money isn't the only important thing we have to give. The Lord asks for our time and talents as well. Remember the parable of the talents? It interests me that the servant who had two talents and magnified them into two more received the same accolades from his lord as the one who was working with five talents. I have no doubt that if the servant with the one talent had magnified that one into just one more, he would have gotten the same reward. And if the servant with the five talents had buried them, don't you think he would have been cast out, even though he would still have had more talents than anyone when the counting was done?

I'm encouraged that the reward is the same for all who are faithful, even though the talents are different. It makes me think that the Lord doesn't need me to be anyone other than who I am. I don't need to carry the tremendous stress of trying to do things the same way someone else would do them. What he *does* ask is that I become the very best me that I can.

I'm thankful for this, because I'm pretty sure that my own best me looks quite different from a lot of other women I know. For example, I'm convinced that if OSHA did home inspections, I would likely be the first woman ever to be issued a lifetime restriction from using a hot-glue gun. I have been known to drape melted glue across the kitchen like crepe paper for a child's birthday party. Strings of it seem to follow me everywhere whenever I fire up that little appliance. I have been the grateful recipient of pinecone wreaths, dainty Christmastree ornaments, and many other products of the hot-glue gun, but I have never mastered the technique of its use myself.

The list of talents that I don't have would fill many pages. But focusing on those is a recipe for despair and stress. I choose to spend that energy instead on figuring out how to magnify the talents I do have. How do I do that? How do two talents get to be four, or five talents grow to be ten?

The answer is very simple. Talents grow when you use them, and they grow the most when you use them in the service of the Lord (which is to say, in the service of your fellow beings—see Mosiah 2:17). Suppose, for example, that you have a talent for baking cookies. It doesn't seem like a very great talent to you, but you decide anyway to lay it on the altar and ask Heavenly Father how it might be used to help him. Suppose he inspires you to take a plate of cookies over to Sister A., who has been having a rough week. You take the cookies, and sure enough, Sister A. really needs the boost. You end up sitting with her for an hour or so while she talks through some of her problems, and you promise to sit by her in church next Sunday so she won't feel so alone there. When you and Sister A. walk into sacrament meeting, you notice that Sister B. is sitting alone as well, so you go sit down by her and help her feel welcome. Before you know it, simple cookie baking has blossomed into a talent for friendship and charity and even missionary service. Isn't that neat?

Take a minute right now and write down two talents that you have. And don't tell me you don't have two talents! If you're reading this book, it means you are literate, and that's a talent many people in the world don't possess. So there's one already! If you feel stuck, you might reread your patriarchal blessing and see if you can get some hints there as to what Heavenly Father feels your talents are.

Now, when you have your two talents written down,

write down next to each one what you're going to do this week to consecrate that talent to the Lord. Ask him in prayer to show you where he needs you the most. Then get in there and start playing! The stresses of life will fade in the sweetness of the music you are making when you serve others.

A final thought about playing the music life gives us: Sometimes the score changes in mid-performance, and we end up playing a different piece from the one we expected. How we handle things when they don't turn out the way we thought they would is one of the greatest tests of mortality.

There are several possible responses to the unexpected twists of life. Sometimes, when they are of minor importance, we can laugh them off. I'm thinking of one Christmas season when we were having a musical sacrament meeting, with various numbers from the ward choir and from specially prepared ensemble groups. We were enjoying a performance by a double quartet of men when, as they approached the end of the song, the music two of them were sharing came up a page short. The tune went on, minus the high tenor part, because those two men were shaking so hard in silent laughter that they couldn't sing.

I know how they felt. Once, years ago, our family was invited to sing in sacrament meeting. I was sure we made a touching little tableau as we stood at the pulpit with our five children, Larry holding the baby, and sang "Families Can Be

Together Forever." We seemed to be getting strange looks, though, from many of the people in the congregation. I happened to glance down as we were finishing the first verse, and discovered that our three-year-old was not singing angelically, as I had envisioned, but crouching behind the podium and then springing up like a jack-in-the-box. This sent me into a rather undignified fit of giggles, which touched off the same reaction in the older children, and poor Larry was left to struggle manfully through the second verse by himself. I wasn't sure at that moment if we *wanted* our family to be together forever! But I guess it was a nice little object lesson for the ward members, showing what family life is really like.

Sometimes the bends in the road hold unexpected blessings. The summer I turned eleven, our family traveled to Montreal, Canada, for the World's Fair, Expo '67. I don't remember much about any of the exhibits we saw there. What I remember is riding the metro and one day arriving at the Fair and discovering that we didn't have our entrance passports, so Dad had to go back to the apartment and get them. I don't remember Mom getting cross at all. She kept us occupied playing games and singing rounds for nearly an hour until Dad got back.

I celebrated my birthday in the middle of that week, and my parents had bought for me one of those little Russian nesting dolls. Everyone stood around watching in amazement as doll after doll popped out from its predecessor. The last three weren't even painted with any features at all; they were too small, and so had been painted in solid colors. The tiniest one was pink, and about the size of a grain of rice. No sooner had I lined all the dolls up for everyone to admire when the pink one fell to the floor. We searched on hands and knees for quite a while to no avail. But my parents were determined. They finally took up the corners of the not-quite-wall-to-wall carpeting and carefully lifted them. Sure enough, the little pink pellet fell to the center of the rug as we all cheered.

I loved the birthday present my parents bought for me. But today, I cherish even more the feeling of being so totally loved by them that they would go the second and third mile to make sure I was happy. They didn't rail over my stupidity for dropping the doll. They didn't fill my birthday or that special trip with unpleasant memories and stress, as they might have. They took the music they had been given, and they figured out a way to play it that brought us closer together as a family.

I particularly admire people who manage to go on playing when the music gets complicated. I have watched, speechless with awe, as friends have dealt with difficulties much more severe than forgotten tickets or lost dolls. I have two close friends who have been diagnosed with breast can-cer, for example, and both of them have chosen to play that piece with such skill and faith that I have been immeasur-ably lifted by their example. I know women who have been widowed, women who have lost children, women who have never been able to have children, women who have lived single all their lives, women who have struggled with sor-rows and disappointments and yet kept playing with all their hearts. The stresses were not removed from their lives, but the Lord made the burdens light upon their backs, and he "did strengthen them that they could bear up their burdens with ease, and they did submit cheerfully and with patience to all the will of the Lord" (Mosiah 24:15). My greatest wish is that I may have that kind of strength, to take whatever music life gives me and, with the Lord's help, make a beautiful melody out of it.

CHAPTER ELEVEN

Don't Clean the Kitchen in Your White Pants

I never buy light-colored pants, mostly because they don't create the hip-diminishing illusion that I get with black or navy blue. But when my husband brought home a pair of white summer pants for me, and they were actually long enough—or as close as I can get, off the rack—I succumbed to their breezy charm. They were so light and cool and fun, I just couldn't resist them.

The problem was, I wasn't used to wearing light pants. One day, I had dug in and was really working "in the zone" to get my kitchen cleaned up when I looked down and it occurred to me in one of those blinding flashes of the obvious that I should not have undertaken that task while wearing my white pants. I know this will seem like a "duh" sort of realization to most, but it hit me too late. I simply hadn't been thinking. Those poor pants were never the same.

It strikes me that a lot of the stress in our lives could be eliminated if we paid a little more attention to avoiding such recipes for disaster. Averting a mess or a crisis is usually so much easier and less painful than cleaning up after one.

For years, whenever I served spaghetti, my husband would strip the younger children down to their underwear for dinner. It wasn't elegant, but it was a heck of a lot more practical. We could plop their tomatoey little bodies straight into the tub after the meal, and I wasn't sobbing over stubborn stains down the tummies of their shirts. It was a good system that served us well until they were old enough to handle that kind of meal with only a napkin as a shield.

My cousin taught me, "Never pour more in a child's glass than you're willing to wipe off the floor." That is a principle worth embracing. And it doesn't necessarily apply just to a child's glass, either. I like to have a glass of water on my nightstand to sip on when I'm reading in bed at night, which is practically every night, but I rarely drink it all before I drift off. My husband warned me for months that I was going to knock that glass over in the middle of the night, and I always waved him off, saying, "I'll deal with that when it happens." It did. And I did. So now I keep *half* a glass of water on my nightstand, and I try to drink most of it, and I set it on a little towel so that if it should spill I can take care of it quickly without waking anyone who might be likely to say "I told you so" in rather a grumpy, middle-of-the-night sort of voice.

I have other habits that I know are likely to bring disaster but that I'm still working to conquer in my life. For example, no matter what time our three-hour block of church starts, I am always rushing at the last minute to get ready to go. Doesn't matter if it's 8:59 or 12:59, you'll find me in the bathroom, brushing my teeth or wrapping the last strands of my hair around the curling iron, waving the rest of the family off so we won't *all* be late. You'd think that in twenty-three years of living literally right across the street from the church building, I could have contrived to be on time for sacrament meeting at least a dozen times, but I'm not sure that has happened. I know I was on time once in October, but that was attributable more to our having gone off Daylight Savings Time and forgetting to set our clocks back than to any great resolution on my part.

Another bad habit of mine is my tendency to default to a series of elaborate avoidance behaviors when I'm having a hard time getting down to a task that really needs doing. Just when I really need to be sitting down to pay the bills, a vision of the cluttered top shelf of the cupboard in the kitchen flits into my mind. I cannot shake that image. I must clean that shelf before I can really concentrate on getting those bills paid. Never mind that the shelf has been cluttered in that fashion for a good six months. Never mind that no one but me is even tall enough to reach that shelf, so no one cares if it's cluttered or not. I go in and clean the shelf—and while I'm there, I notice that the shelf paper is getting a bit shabby, and before I know it, I'm happily trimming and pasting and rearranging while my bill-paying deadline is flying past and disaster is looming.

My all-time favorite bumper sticker proclaims, "Warning! Dates on calendar may be closer than they appear!" The older I get, the truer this is. I've learned that the surest way to put my life into lasting overload is to fail to pay attention to things as they come up. If I set something important aside to think about another day, chances are it won't get thought about at all until some nasty notice or phone call yanks it back into the forefront weeks down the road. In the brief periods of my life when I temporarily get control of the procrastination habit (and there have been as many as six or seven of those in twenty-plus years), I'm always a little surprised at how much more I can get done.

Another source of difficulty and potential disaster is lack of knowledge—although I'd like to say, parenthetically, that there is occasionally such a thing as too much knowledge. When I landed in the hospital with toxic shock syndrome two months after the birth of our second child, I made the mistake of sneaking a peek at my hospital chart. I had always wondered what they were writing down there so diligently as they interviewed you, and the nurse had left the folder in my room while she went to check on someone else. So I seized the opportunity to have a look. Well, the admitting nurse had written: "Patient is a cheerful, cooperative, well-informed, overweight white female." I have to admit that "cheerful, cooperative, and well-informed" did not exactly balance out "overweight" on the self-esteem scale at that point in my life. I could never quite look that nurse in the eye the rest of the time I was there.

However, I have been much more likely to be stung by what I didn't know than by what I did. I have been subjected to repeated humiliations, for example, from ward members who remember the year I agreed to cook one of the turkeys for the annual ward Christmas dinner. I had never cooked a turkey before, so I was careful to get detailed instructions from the chairwoman of the activity, but she neglected to tell me that there's a little sack in the bird that contains the giblets and neck and stuff. I proudly toted my beautiful, brown bird over to the ward kitchen, only to meet with peals of laughter from the women who were there cooking the vegetables as they discovered that bag intact in my cooked turkey.

In that case, it really didn't matter. My willingness to cook the turkey in the first place was the important thing, and if I lacked a little know-how, no one was really hurt by it. However, although a lot can be accomplished by a willing soul, there are times when you just plain have to know what you're doing.

I remember attending a mother-daughter Primary party where they were planning to pull taffy, but the Primary president, who was the one who knew how to do it, was unable at the last moment to attend. Undaunted, the leaders forged ahead, and I assured them that I had pulled taffy plenty of times in my childhood, which was true. I didn't really take into account the difference between helping to pull taffy as a child under adult supervision and being in actual charge of the taffy pulling.

The first step, of course, was cooking the taffy, and the leaders had the recipe in hand but, regrettably, no candy thermometer. Not to worry. I knew how to test if candy had reached the hard-ball stage: You drop a little spoonful of it into a cup of cold water, and if it readily forms into a ball, you're there. What I didn't remember was that you need to take the pan of candy off the burner while you're testing it, so that it doesn't continue to cook. Unbeknownst to us, while we were ruminating over the little blob in the bottom of the cup, the taffy in the pan was boiling itself up to hard-crack stage.

When we finally decided that the candy was indeed

ready, the women turned to me. After all, I had known how to test the candy. I must be an expert in what to do next. Did I admit that it had been thirty years since I had been involved in taffy creation, and that I had never been the head cook in any candy-making incident? No, I blundered right on ahead. At home we had always poured the hot taffy out onto a buttered marble slab. In the absence of marble, I suggested that we just butter the wooden butcher block in the center of the kitchen and pour it onto that.

In hindsight, I can see why that was a really bad idea. For one thing, you pour candy out onto marble to cool it. Wood has this heat-retaining capacity that just cooks the candy even more. It also has lots of little pores and cracks into which hot melted sugar can run.

Things seemed to be going forward smoothly enough until the candy began to cool. By the time it was cool enough to begin pulling, it was starting to get hard. The girls complained, but I told them they just needed to work the air into it. We proceeded with buttered fingers, but only a small portion of the blob on the counter was claimed.

After half an hour or so of mostly fruitless pulling, we let the girls off the hook and agreed to throw the mess away. Regrettably, by then the remainder of the unpulled taffy had basically fused itself to the wooden countertop like a coat of polyurethane. We couldn't pry it off with our fingers or spatulas. We tried chiseling it off with kitchen knives; some of it yielded, but only an inch at a time. We finally resorted to dumping boiling water onto it to melt it. It took forever. I was not a very popular woman by the end of the party, and I had certainly lost any credibility as a candy maker!

Everyone would have been a lot happier that night if I had not pretended to know what I was doing. Maybe we would have called a real expert for advice. At the very least, we might have abandoned the taffy in the pan instead of on the counter, which would have made for a ten-minute cleanup instead of a two-hour fiasco.

So I'm a real proponent of avoiding potential disasters. In that spirit, here are a few other pieces of miscellaneous advice that I'm happy to pass along in the interest of helping to prevent accidents before they happen.

1. If you need a breath mint in order to face a social situation, be sure you consume it completely before you have to use your voice. I popped an Altoids in my mouth during a choir warm-up once, and ingested it right into my lung. I thought I was going to die. There I was, trying to be inconspicuous, hacking little coughs of curiously strong peppermint breath for about five minutes before one particularly powerful cough propelled the mint out of my lung and across the room. Bad breath probably would have been a less embarrassing alternative.

2. If you're going to take your children to a pond or park somewhere, and feeding the ducks is on the itinerary, save that activity for when you're just about ready to go home. Then be ready to jump in your car the moment you run out of bread crumbs. A pleasant experience can turn quickly into a nightmare when a bunch of hungry waterfowl take off after a child who has run out of crusts. This is especially true if there are any geese in the mix. Geese are mean.

3. If you're helping a group of people tie a quilt, and someone on the other side of the quilt needs the scissors, don't try to slide the scissors across the quilt to that person. Pick them up and hand them around. It's really easy for the tip of the blade to catch and slice into the quilt, and if you have to put a patch on that rip you will be reminded of your stupidity every night for the next two decades.

4. Zucchini is not like corn. Unless you really, really, *really* love zucchini, or have a ready market for it outside your own neighborhood, do not plant two full rows of it in your garden.

5. Don't microwave hot chocolate after you've already put the mix in the water.

6. If you put the elders quorum in charge of cooking the ward dinner, make sure they're also in charge of cleaning up afterward. Or at least warn whoever *is* going to be cleaning

up afterward, so they can line the oven bottom with foil and spread newspapers on the kitchen floor.

7. If you're going to let a two-year-old lick the chocolate frosting off the beaters, put him in his high chair to do it. Do not let him range freely through the house. And take off his clothes, if it's not too cold.

8. Do not, under any circumstances, have a permanent marker in a house where any of the inhabitants are under five years of age. Do not imagine you can hide it away from their prying eyes. They will find it. They will use it. You will have to repaint.

9. If you have long hair, don't lean over the sewing machine too closely. It can pick up a strand and jerk your whole head into the machine. Don't get too close to the candles on your birthday cake, either.

10. Don't say any words in front of a toddler that you don't want to hear coming out of his mouth at Grandma's house or in nursery.

11. If you're working on your weight, don't wear one of those belts that has a buckle-type center but no holes in the belt and no latch to feed through a hole to secure it. That kind of belt has a nasty tendency to pop open when you bend or stoop, and having a four-year-old cry out for the whole Primary to hear, "Uh-oh, better skinny up!" is not a big self-esteem booster.

12. If there's a stray sock on the floor when you're vacuuming, stop and pick it up. Don't try to nudge it out of the way with the nozzle of the vacuum.

13. Don't get so entrenched in the habit of flipping up your skirt to adjust your half-slip that you accidentally do it on the way out of sacrament meeting.

14. While we're on the subject of lingerie, don't be lulled into a false sense of security by a black slip. It is easier than you might think to forget you haven't put your skirt on yet.

15. Unless you want to make it a permanent part of your wardrobe, don't affix one of those "Hello, My Name Is . . ." tags to a suede jacket.

16. If your recipe calls for salt, don't measure it over the mixing bowl, especially if there are toddlers climbing up your legs at the time.

17. It's perfectly all right to serve macaroni and cheese to the children if you and your husband are going out for the evening. It's also all right to ask them to put their plates in the dishwasher when they're finished. But if you're going to ask them to run the dishwasher after they've loaded it, be sure they know the difference between *dish* soap and *dishwasher* soap.

18. To clean a truckload of suds off your kitchen floor, scoop up as many of the bubbles as you can with a pail and

pile them in the bathtub. Then turn on the shower for a few minutes. Work barefoot!

19. Leaving a toddler and a large, open jar of peanut butter alone in the same room, even for five minutes, is not a good idea—particularly if the toddler has been watching you wallpaper his bedroom recently.

Most important of all, remember to laugh! Some disasters simply can't be foreseen or averted, no matter how vigilant you are. Life is a messy game. Play smart when you can, but if you lose a point or two along the way, don't panic. Experts say we learn best from our mistakes. I like to think that makes me pretty smart!

CHAPTER TWELVE

Read to the End of the Story

After attending an all-day conference plus an evening performance at Brigham Young University, I was tired and ready to go home. I wasn't exactly looking forward to the forty-five-minute drive ahead of me, but I was extremely happy at the prospect of not walking anymore. I had hauled my carcass from one end of campus to another and all around in between until I thought my muscles would just plain go on strike. It was all I could do to stagger to my car, but an extra shot of adrenaline spurred by the dark night and the lonely parking lot helped me along, and I collapsed gratefully into the driver's seat and just rested for a few moments before buckling up and starting the motor.

I don't know why arrows painted on the pavement of parking lots have to be so darn confusing. In my attempts to find the exit, I circled past the same landmarks a couple of times, but I finally spotted the gate ahead and manuevered toward it. The only problem was, the gate was closed. I didn't have a card or anything to insert in a slot, which was immaterial, since there didn't seem to be a slot anyway. I crept a little closer, hoping to see a help box with a button on it somewhere. Nothing. "Great," I thought, "I've parked in a daytime lot, and now it's closed, and I'll be stuck here until tomorrow morning. Now I'm going to have to call Larry and drag him out in the middle of the night to drive down to Provo and pick me up so I don't have to spend the stupid night in my car . . ." All this time I was grumbling to myself, I was inching closer to the gate. Just as I was about to back up and drive back around to a parking space so I could find a phone, the gate opened all by itself! Apparently, it was set up like an automatic door at the supermarket, to open when the customer breaks the light beam at a certain point on the way to the door. I drove on through, feeling pretty sheepish, and headed for home.

I wonder how many opportunities in my life I have for-feited because the gate ahead seemed closed to me. How many times have I assumed that I just wasn't talented enough or smart enough or beautiful enough even to try? How many gates might have opened if I had just had the courage and the faith to keep moving forward?

I like to see where I'm going, to know that all the gates work and that I'm supposed to be going through them. It is particularly trying for me not to know how things are going to work out. But I'm happy to be able to say that, at one crucial time in my life, I had the faith to keep walking even though the pathway was not very clear.

I was in my first year of college, enrolled as an elementary education major, when one day I was struck forcibly by the thought that I didn't want to teach school. This was a shock to me; I had planned to be a teacher for as long as I could remember. I had taught Primary and Junior Sunday School for several years and was volunteering as a Cub Scout leader in an underprivileged area of town. Who knows, maybe some of the experiences I had had to that point were trying to tell me something. As much as I loved children, maybe I didn't have the patience for a whole flock of them at once over the course of a full school year. Whatever the reasons, the more I thought about it, the clearer it was to me that I wasn't cut out to be an elementary school teacher.

This left me with rather a hole in my plans. If I wasn't going to major in elementary education, what *should* I major in? Casting my mind over my high school years, I had to admit that the courses I had really enjoyed the most were my English classes. However, as firmly as I knew I did not want to teach elementary school, I knew with an even greater certainty that I didn't want to teach English on any level. What on earth would I do with a degree in English?

This question was prevalent not just in my mind but in the minds and on the lips of many family members and friends over the next two years. My parents, to their credit, never discouraged me from pursuing an English major, but I'm sure they must have wondered where it would take me. Some others were not so supportive; when they heard I wasn't even applying for a teaching certificate, they snorted and suggested not too kindly that I was wasting my time and would be sorry down the road.

I didn't know how to explain it, but I liked majoring in English. It *felt* good. I enjoyed writing papers and taking essay tests and reading, reading, reading. I especially loved a series of classes I took in oral interpretation of literature, where the basic goal was to demonstrate your understanding of the story or the poem by the way you read it to the class. So I went blissfully along, undecided clear through my junior year about what I would do when I finished my degree but still feeling inexplicably calm about my decision.

The summer before my senior year, I received a letter in the mail about a new magazine that was going to be started over at the LDS Institute of Religion, one that would hopefully serve as a bridge between the LDS students and the rest of the student body. The letter was an invitation being sent to all English and journalism majors to "audition" to serve on the staff of the magazine. I thought that might be kind of fun, so I sent in my application, went in for an interview, and was surprised to be asked, a few weeks later, to become the magazine's associate editor.

In the process of that little assignment, which grew when the editor resigned midyear, leaving me in charge of the whole publication, I learned that I had skills that might actually be marketable. I mean, I knew I was a good speller—I was always picking out errors on billboards and menus—but it had never crossed my mind that there might be people willing to pay me for pointing out their mistakes.

The happy ending to this story is that I graduated from college and sent out resumes just in time to be hired onto the editorial staff at Deseret Book Company when they needed help working on the new LDS edition of the King James Version of the Bible. I had found a career that was satisfying, suited to my skills, and of value in building up the Lord's kingdom. What's more, I could pursue it part time at home, staying there with my five children until they were old enough to go to school, and then pick it back up again full time when the season was right for that.

Majoring in English was the best possible choice I could have made. I just needed to hang on long enough to find out why.

President Gordon B. Hinckley often says, "Things will work out." That seems to be true more often than not. The hard part is all the stuff in the middle that's happening while things are moving toward that working-out point. The happy ending is not always easy to see.

I remember an evening when my husband and I, newly-weds without children of our own yet, had gone with my cousins and their little ones to a drive-in movie. We had gotten there while it was still light, and it seemed to be taking the sun an interminably long time to sink, so I was attempting to entertain the children with a lively recounting of "Rapunzel," the first fairy tale that occurred to me when someone suggested a storytelling time.

I think the Brothers Grimm were aptly named, because if you're familiar at all with the original versions of some of those old fairy tales, you know they're mighty grim. Cinderella's stepsister, for instance, actually gets her foot into the glass slipper by cutting off her toes, a fact conveyed to the prince by a bird chirping in his ear as he's on the way back to the castle with the imposter in his carriage. In "Rapunzel," the hapless prince is hurled from the tower by the wicked witch and has his eyes scratched out in a briar patch. I haven't seen the recently released *Rapunzel Barbie* video, but I suspect that little scene is omitted from that particular recounting. I, however, was proceeding in fine form and telling that portion of the story with great relish when I noticed the eyes of the children opening wider and wider in horror. Tears were just surfacing when my cousin hissed, "Get to the end! Jump to the end of the story!" So I threw the climax to the wind and rushed through the part where Rapunzel gets banished to the wilderness and bears twin babies, hurrying ahead to the point where the wandering, blind prince hears her singing and staggers to her side, and her tears fall onto his eye sockets and restore his sight. The children's weeping turned quickly to tears of relief as the prince and Rapunzel lived happily ever after in the end.

I'm not sure those original fairy tales needed to be quite so graphic—in fact, I'm quite sure they did not—but one thing I can agree with: A good story needs conflict. So does a good mortal life. As Lehi expressed it: "It must needs be, that there is an opposition in all things." Why? "To bring about [God's] eternal purposes in the end of man. . . . Wherefore, the Lord God gave unto man that he should act for himself. Wherefore, man could not act for himself save it should be that he was enticed by the one or the other" (2 Nephi 2:11, 15–16). Agency, one of the vital eternal principles over which the great war in heaven was waged, is dependent upon choice, which implies the possibility of choosing wrongly. The propensity of the natural man toward those wrong choices is amply demonstrated in the history of the world or in the behavior in the corridors of any middle school in the country.

When we're stuck in the "conflict-rich" part of our life's story, it's hard to keep believing in the happy ending. It helps to keep track of some of the interim happy endings we've experienced, times when we've actually made it through some tunnels that seemed to have no light at their ends.

For example, our oldest daughter, when she was a teenager, had a series of unfortunate and somewhat freakish automobile incidents that resulted in our insurance carrier dropping her from our policy. The premiums on the proffered "high-risk" policy were more than we could handle at the time, and knowing that she would be heading off to school in the fall, where she wouldn't even have access to a car, we elected simply to not allow her to drive for the summer.

A sociable person with many friends who had access to cars, our daughter accepted this decision with reasonably good grace—until her search for a summer job led her to a place in Sandy, several miles south of our home. Sticking to our guns, we obtained bus and light-rail schedules and worked out the routes with her. It was a pain, really. She had to catch a bus to the light-rail station, take the light-rail train almost to the end of the line, and hop on another bus to get up to her work location. The first week, she was in tears. The stop for the bus she needed wasn't at the place designated on the printed schedule, and she ended up walking over a mile in the afternoon heat to get to the light-rail station. She missed connections easily and was late for work a couple of times. The whole thing seemed almost impossibly complicated.

Unfortunately, she had no choice. She couldn't afford the $150 a month for insurance, so she had to work out the alternative transportation or give up the job. No one was surprised that by the end of the second week she had it down pat. She was completely self-sufficient that summer for her transportation needs and ended up actually enjoying the challenge of getting where she wanted to go.

A couple of years later, when that same daughter ended up in Zimbabwe on her mission, she was grateful for the skills she had developed at getting around. A walk to the light-rail station on nice cement sidewalks seems like a cinch compared to her now-regular treks on the dusty roads of Africa. The strength she has gained through conquering small trials has served her well as the trials have gotten bigger, and each successfully navigated challenge gives her increased courage for the next one.

We see this pattern in the scriptures as well, when prophets often point to past successes as reasons for current hope. Witness Alma, reminding the people of Zarahemla of the miraculous deliverance of their fathers from bondage (see Alma 5:3–5). Nephi, persuading his brothers to try again to obtain the brass plates after two unsuccessful attempts, evoked the example of Moses parting the Red Sea to awaken their faith (see 1 Nephi 4:2–3).

As Lehi pointed out, "All things have been done in the wisdom of him who knoweth all things" (2 Nephi 2:24). The road to deliverance often winds through several varieties of plagues along its course. I try to think of such times as "spiritual aerobics," a grueling but necessary mortal workout that will help us develop the spiritual muscle we need to be valiant servants of the Lord.

While serving his mission in North Carolina, my son had an experience that I think illustrates this principle. He and his companion were tracting in an area that was not too heavily populated, with about one house every quarter-mile or so, and fields in between. As they were walking from house to house one day, they noticed a pack of dogs in a field as they passed, but the dogs just looked at them and didn't come any closer, so the elders proceeded on and went to the door of the house nearby. They had no sooner gotten onto the porch when the four pit bulls careened out of the field and came after them. One of them was biting my son on the leg, and he was beating it off with his scriptures and shouting while his companion stood frozen. Finally the woman of the house came to the door and called off the dogs. With typical missionary understatement, my son wrote, "She wasn't too interested in the gospel, so we left."

Then the full force of what had happened suddenly hit him. "I looked down at my shredded, slobbered-on church pants, and I started to cry," he wrote. "But the dog's teeth didn't go through my 'armor,' and I know the Lord was protecting me."

Now, I'm pretty sure that as a mother I had prayed more than once that my missionary son would be able to learn that the Lord would be with him even when times got rough. Sending him into the jaws of pit bulls was not exactly the method I would have chosen in order to confirm that message! But even at that, I can see the miracle in four pit bulls charging but only one attacking. I can see the miracle in shredded pants but unbroken skin. I can see the miracle in a young man learning in a most dramatic way that "all things shall work together for good to them that walk uprightly" (D&C 100:15).

All things. Not just the happy ones, like seminary graduation and snowboarding with friends and getting to pick your favorite dinner on your birthday. The hard times, the soul-searing experiences, the apparently senseless things that sock you right in the jaw when you least expect it, those too can work for your good. Don't misunderstand me—I don't think there's anything good about pain itself. But pain working in the life of a good person can be turned to meaningful purpose because the Lord, whose ways are not our ways, has promised to make it so.

Our wise Father in heaven doesn't always remove the pit bulls from our lives. As much as we wish it were otherwise, we are always going to have conflict. "What can't be cured must be endured," says a chirpy character from a novel I read in my childhood that I can't remember the title of now.

I've always kind of hated that word *endure*. To me, it conjures up a long haul through a desert wasteland, or hanging on by your fingernails when you're about to slide down a cliff. We're admonished often to "endure to the end," and although I recognize the importance of that, it has still always sounded tedious and even unfulfilling to me.

Then one day I saw a commercial for an anniversary diamond ring, and the tag line said something about "an enduring gift" along with the "diamonds are forever" slogan. It put a new twist on that word *enduring* for me. I began to think of it as something lasting and bright and strong. I pictured that diamond twinkling against a dull gray background (effective marketing on the part of the jewelry guys) and thought, "That's what I want to be." I want to shine even when the world is dark. I want to outlast all the grayness of my mortal trials. I want to leave an inheritance of faith and courage that my children after me can pass down, like a diamond ring, from generation to generation.

So now, when people speak of "enduring to the end," I think instead, "*Be* enduring to the end. Be strong, and bright, and radiant. Let people know that you will always believe in the happy ending to the story—because the story doesn't end here."

Some happy endings will never be read in this life. But the atonement of Jesus Christ promises us that our stories will all have successful conclusions one day, if we put our trust in him. He who sees the end from the beginning and desires above all for us to enjoy immortality and eternal life will lead us to our own "happily ever afters," if we will follow in his ways. Things may not always make sense. Gates may be closed to us for a time. And trials may assail us. But if we can be enduring to the end, all these things will work for our good, and we will find ourselves as polished gems in the hands of our Maker.

ABOUT THE AUTHOR

Emily Watts is a lover of words. She is a graduate of the University of Utah and has been an editor at Deseret Book Company for more than twenty years, where she continues to serve as Assistant Director of Publishing. Her first book, *Being the Mom: 10 Coping Strategies I Learned by Accident Because I Had Children on Purpose,* remains very popular and in a natural way spawned this second book. A frequent speaker at events of interest to women, a wife, and a mother of five children, Emily is herself a "really busy woman." She is married to Larry Watts, and they live in Salt Lake City.